Approaches to Ethics

For Butterworth-Heinemann:

Commissioning Editor: Mary Seager
Project Development Manager: Catherine Jackson
Project Manager: Morven Dean
Design: George Ajayi

Approaches to Ethics

Nursing Beyond Boundaries

Edited by

Verena Tschudin RN RM DipCouns BSc(Hons) MA PhD
University of Surrey, UK

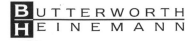

BUTTERWORTH
HEINEMANN

EDINBURGH LONDON NEW YORK OXFORD PHILADELPHIA ST LOUIS SYDNEY TORONTO 2003

BUTTERWORTH-HEINEMANN
An imprint of Elsevier Science Limited

First published 2003

ISBN 0 7506 5326 4

British Library Cataloguing in Publication Data
A catalogue record for this book is available from the British Library

Library of Congress Cataloguing in Publication Data
A catalog record for this book is available from the Library of
Congress

Notice
Medical knowledge is constantly changing. Standard safety
precautions must be followed, but as new research and clinical
experience broaden our knowledge, changes in treatment and drug
therapy may become necessary or appropriate. Readers are advised to
check the most current product information provided by the
manufacturer of each drug to be administered to verify the
recommended dose, the method and duration of administration, and
contraindications. It is the responsibility of the practitioner, relying on
experience and knowledge of the patient, to determine dosages and
the best treatment for each individual patient. Neither the Publisher
nor the author assumes any liability for any injury and/or damage to
persons or property arising from this publication.

The Publisher

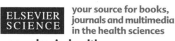 your source for books,
journals and multimedia
in the health sciences
www.elsevierhealth.com

The
publisher's
policy is to use
**paper manufactured
from sustainable forests**

Printed in China
C/01

Contents

Contributors

Wendy Austin
I am a Professor in Nursing at the University of Alberta, specialising in psychiatric/mental health nursing. I was an advisor in mental health to the International Council of Nurses and am a former President of the Canadian Federation of Mental Health Nurses. In my research work I explore mainly a relational approach to ethical issues in mental health care.

Ann Begley
I have been teaching health care ethics for some years and have learned that professional ethics requires more than knowledge of theory or rule following. Sensitivity to the perspectives of clients and colleagues is crucial. This can be fostered in the inexperienced and enhanced in the experienced practitioner by tapping into the insight offered by such media as literature and films.

Vangie Bergum
I am currently Director of the John Dossetor Health Ethics Centre and Professor of Nursing at the University of Alberta. My work in health ethics began with doctoral research on the experience of mothering. I believe that ethical dialogue needs an interdisciplinary focus because issues of ethical action cross the borders of disciplines.

Anne Davis
During 34 years at the University of California, San Francisco, I established the nursing ethics programme, served as a member of the Clinical Ethics Committee and the Research Ethics Committee, and numerous other positions. I have visited 115 countries and worked in the Middle East, Africa, India and China. Since 1995, I have been Professor at Nagano College of Nursing, Japan. My major research interests are end-of-life issues and international nursing ethics.

John Dossetor
As a UK physician, I became an early Canadian nephrologist responsible for a kidney transplant programme at McGill from 1963. I moved to the University of Alberta in 1969 to continue research in clinical transplant immunology. In 1985 I made a 13-year-long career change to health ethics. Since 1998 I have lived in Ottawa, enjoying retirement.
Wendy Austin adds: John's leadership was responsible for the creation of the John Dossetor Health Ethics Centre. In 1995 he was awarded the Order of Canada.

Helen Graham
I am currently the manager of the Inpatient and Outpatient Cardiac Rehabilitation Program at Penrose-St Francis Healthcare Services in Colorado Springs, Colorado. I am also a Nursing PhD candidate at the University of Colorado Health Science Center in Denver, Colorado. My focus of study is on long-term outcomes of cardiac rehabilitation. My goal post-dissertation is to study programme effectiveness through the use of relational narratives.

Sandy Haegert
A lecturer/tutor at the Western Cape College of Nursing now, I was a Senior Nurse Education/Manager for Islington and Ipswich Health Authorities from 1978 to 1989. I presently teach South African nursing students (of all races and mainly seniors) ethos and professional practice, including ethics. I have taught psychology, philosophy and sociology, including culture, at all levels.

Joan Liaschenko
My work as a dually appointed Associate Professor at the Center for Bioethics and School of Nursing has me doing the expected— teaching ethics in the School of Nursing, and sometimes the unexpected—teaching ethics in the School of Veterinary Medicine. Maybe my six cats had something to do with this. I believe in the necessity of interdisciplinary ethics education and the value of the humanities for understanding ourselves and the world.

Robin Lindsay
I studied nursing in Utah and Colorado, and practised all over the USA and Western Europe while an army wife. My interest is in community health care of populations, but I have enjoyed working as a family nurse practitioner, as a telephone triage nurse, and in establishing a paediatric clinic in a rural native Indian town. I like to read, play the flute and hike, and am a Harry Potter fan for its therapeutic value.

Helen Oppenheimer
MA(Oxon), DD(Lambeth). As a child I had two ambitions: to have a family and to write books. These still matter most to me. My husband and I met at Oxford. We now live in Jersey and have three married daughters and ten grandchildren. My books endeavour to explain a credible Christian faith. The latest is *Making Good: Creation, Tragedy and Hope* (SCM Press).

Elizabeth Peter
I am currently an Assistant Professor in the Faculty of Nursing and a member of the Joint Centre for Bioethics at the University of Toronto. During my early years of graduate education, my discovery of feminist scholarship helped me to understand how nursing work became devalued and to envision a better future for nursing. Today, feminist ethics informs both my research and my teaching. The completion of this chapter with Joan Liaschenko further demonstrates to me the significance of friendship, a deeply held feminist ideal.

Maj-Britt Råholm
My great sources of inspiration are classical music and the wonderful island of Crete in the Aegean Sea. I am a Principal Lecturer at Vaasa Polytechnic, Department of Social and Health Care. My primary research interest focuses on the experiences of suffering and the ethics of care surrounding coronary artery bypass surgery.

P Anne Scott
I am a Professor and Head of School, Dublin City University. I have worked clinically and as an academic in Ireland, Scotland and Kenya. My interest in health care ethics was first sparked during my undergraduate preparation in philosophy. One of my core research interests is the virtues and clincal practice, and links between the arts and health care.

Verena Tschudin
Having started as a nurse and moved through counselling to ethics, my main work now is as Editor of the international journal *Nursing Ethics*. I have a part-time teaching position at the University of Surrey. Writing has been both a job and a joy for over 20 years.

Stan van Hooft
I teach philosophy at Deakin University in Australia. I have done all the usual academic things, including writing books on caring and on critical thinking for nurses, but my main love is to facilitate Socratic dialogues in various settings and to conduct a monthly 'Philosophy Café' in a Melbourne bookshop.

Preface

Not much in life is certain nowadays. Perhaps this is why people have become more interested in ethics as one means of indicating right and wrong. Nowhere is this more evident than in politics and health care. Since these two areas are closely related in the UK, where free state health care still applies, nurses and midwives in particular have had to think and work ethically, and they have had to learn fast.

When faced with the need for curriculum development and strategies to teach students in ethics, many nurses turned to the sources they could obtain easily. These tended to be texts on medical ethics, often heavy with theories and principles. When applying these texts to nursing, the word 'medical' was simply crossed out and 'nursing' written in its place. On the whole, for the last two decades of the twentieth century, nurses worked with materials that were at best not ideally suited to nursing and at worst denied nursing any credibility. Many situations were explained from the starting point of a principle or a theory, sometimes desperately trying to fit round pegs into square holes. Many of us were put into lecture theatres holding up to 200 students, to talk about and try to understand 'confidentiality' or some such vital subject, without the possibility of any realistic interchange. Thankfully, for students and lecturers alike, better ways are now emerging.

Because much is demanded in and of ethics, the subject itself is changing and widening, and so is its learning, reasoning, body of knowledge and teaching. This book is witness to this change. Its collection of original chapters and reprinted articles is only one way of saying: 'There is more to ethics than the obvious, the safe, the well known, what "they" think or say, or what might be expected.'

My original intention was to publish a 'reader' of articles that had first appeared in the journal *Nursing Ethics*, consisting of examples of various approaches to ethics. To my surprise and delight, most of the authors I approached about reprinting their work immediately proposed to write original chapters; some even said they would write two! Thus the project became different and more 'engaged', which is in itself an indication of a new approach to ethics.

The approaches to ethics represented here are some of the most well known and popular, but they are by no means the only ones. Indeed, it is right that new ones should emerge and develop. The significant trend at the moment is to stress and strengthen relationships between people at every level. Within nursing, the nurse–patient relationship has always had a strong place, but, considered from the standpoint of ethics, it becomes the crucial element. When feminist ethics first became established, it seemed to demand almost a complete rethinking of ethics, because starting with something as intangible and unstable as a relationship was almost like turning history upside down. Ethics had been built on the idea that logic and reason alone were capable of making decisions. Accepting that 'touchy-feely' things like relationships could also be the bases for legitimate ethical decisions needed courage. This courage has been proved not only right but the necessary balance. This is especially so in health care, where patients start off in a vulnerable position because of illness and suffering, and reaching them where they are by means of a relationship may be the only way of showing respect and acceptance. It is therefore not surprising that different ways of working with and expressing the relationship have become more clarified and clearly expressed.

Even if some authors contributing to this volume treat the same subject, they do it in different ways. Ethics is not simply about abstract ideas, but about how to get on with each other in daily life. Thus, individuality matters, and this is shown in these authors' way of engaging with and addressing readers, thus also forming a relationship. The chapters are written from a point of sharing, not teaching. The authors are not declaring that their own way of doing and thinking is either right or superior, but they are giving indications that the elements they describe can be helpful in understanding actions and situations. In relationships it is vital that we should understand and respect each other. Anything that helps us to do that is therefore welcome.

All nursing practice is ethical practice. Even how we say 'good morning' to a patient counts, and to patients it matters how they are treated. It even matters how they are given a cup of tea: do the cup and saucer match? If not, why not? Nursing practice is excellent (one criterion for it being ethical practice) only when practitioners are able to make good professional decisions, based on experience and knowledge, and with the expertise of judging the outcomes. This demands reflection on and in practice, and this is where the various approaches to ethics come into their own. They are able to guide reflection, highlight aspects of practice, philosophy, tradition, culture and needs, and help to shape arguments and values that are pointing beyond the immediate situation, but starting from it.

The greater freedom of using different approaches can be confusing to some people. Is it possible to acknowledge ethics as something that guides and directs, when there are so many ways to do this? Ethics is only the means to get to somewhere, it is not the way. It is like a

signpost, not the path. Ethics is a description of what happens between people, not what individuals are. The person 'does' ethics, and that can only be guided, or addressed, or awoken. This is what some of these approaches point to. It is the individual who takes the responsibility for behaving in a certain way, but that way can be influenced by pointing out certain aspects of how actions and behaviour become more adequate or wholesome. Thus, it is not only right to have different approaches, it is necessary.

The chapters that highlight different cultural approaches make a valid point in this direction. Personal and family values give us a sense of belonging, but the cultural values define us in a wider setting. With so much more travel and movement of people around the world, not only do health care professionals have to learn about the norms and values of other people, they can themselves benefit from the insights that others have, and apply them to their own setting and culture. It is not a question of amalgamating them, or labelling them as either 'good' or 'better' (thus saying that others are 'bad' or 'worse'), but of trying to understand the essence of some other values, perhaps in order to understand one's own from a new or different angle. It is remarkable that, when we really listen to other people's stories, we hear our own in them, differently expressed perhaps, and therefore refreshing the understanding of our own values. Two simple examples are the concept of 'ubuntu' in Sandy Haegert's chapter. Ubuntu can be translated variously, but one way is: 'I am a person because you are a person.' When 'love your neighbour as your self' is considered closely, these two expressions are remarkably similar, but in their concepts enhance each other. In my own chapter I relate the story of Monkey, who had sneakily eaten the peaches of eternal life. Does this not sound remarkably similar to Adam and Eve who had eaten the forbidden apple of the knowledge between good and evil? We need not seek the differences or similarities, but to understand what the stories point us to. They point us to deeper connection with ourselves and others, and how to respect and foster these connections in respect. The stories of eating forbidden fruit are one way of indicating what ethics is about: making the right or fitting choices, because we have to live with the consequences for a long time.

There is no single ethical approach that is valid everywhere for everyone. It is not necessary and would not be workable. What we need is practitioners who can listen and engage with each other, and with their clients and patients, in such a way that they foster ethical thinking and behaviour. To do this, we need above all integrity, which stems as much out of self-knowledge as out of knowledge of the other.

When we are in touch with both, we can celebrate diversity and otherness.

The approaches presented here are a selection of some of those used regularly in nursing. There are and will be others. Perhaps some readers work with others, or will formulate others in due course. The essence of different approaches is not that they work for one person, or are one person's good ideas, but that they are applicable widely, and are based on need and contribute to the wider good. This book aims to make a contribution to all of these.

London 2003   V.T.

Caring and ethics in nursing

Stan van Hooft

This opening chapter is by a well-known writer on caring and ethics in nursing. Stan van Hooft has written and lectured extensively in this field. He details how caring is a virtue, and how virtue is necessary to caring, a topic that has often been discussed from different angles and with different emphases. Readers could therefore be forgiven for thinking that they have read it all before. However, Stan writes with a freshness that never fails to surprise, even on a familiar topic. This careful analysis of the topic of caring and ethics in the light of virtue is therefore particularly welcome and will inspire further thought and, indeed, real practical caring that is also deeply ethical.

INTRODUCTION

It is now a commonplace that a central concept used in the description of nursing practice is that of caring. The work of Patricia Benner (Benner and Wrubel 1989), Jean Watson (1985, 1988), Madeline Leininger (1981, 1988), Simone Roach (1992, 1997) and others has been at the forefront of pushing to have this concept accepted into the mainstream of nursing studies. Moreover, such feminist writers as Sara Fry (1989) and Peta Bowden (1997) have used the notion of caring to articulate what is distinctive about nursing as a profession dominated by women. A significant body of writing has also emerged in order to explore what the concept means in practical terms or when it is operationalised (Wallis 1998, Wilkes and Wallis 1993). Furthermore, there continues to be philosophical and conceptual inquiry into the meaning of the concept, both in the context of nursing and in more general terms (Blustein 1991, van Hooft 1995). There has, however, also been criticism (Allmark 1995, Hanford 1994, Kuhse 1997, Nelson 1992). In order to show how polarised the consequent debate has been, here are two striking and characteristic quotes:

As an expression of nursing, caring is the intentional and authentic presence of the nurse with another who is recognized as person living caring and growing in caring. Here, the nurse endeavors to come to know the other as caring person and seeks to understand how that person might be supported, sustained, and strengthened in their unique process of living caring and growing in caring. (Boykin and Schoenhofer 1993, p. 25)

In contrast:

Expecting contemporary health care professionals to care for their patients is as unreasonable as expecting love from a prostitute. In both cases, the relationship seems intimate, but the exchange of money, the infrequency of contact, and the one-dimensionality of the relationship makes the relationship purely professional. Emotional attachment is incidental and destructive to the practice. (Curzer 1993, p. 66)

I take these quotes to be representative of two antithetical concepts of caring in nursing. I will call the first the 'emotional concept' and the second the 'behavioural concept'. The emotional concept stresses the feelings of concern and relationship between nurse and patient that should inspire and motivate professional caring practice, while the behavioural concept focuses on the effective performance of professional caring practices, whether or not they are motivated by feelings of sympathy or rapport.

Rather than re-entering the debate that this dichotomy highlights, I wish to correlate them with two differing concepts of ethics. I want to suggest that the emotional concept aligns with what has become known as a 'caring perspective' in ethics, while the behavioural concept is more in tune with a 'justice perspective'.

What are these differing perspectives in ethics? The research of Carol Gilligan (1982) has demonstrated the centrality of caring, conceived as a distinctly feminine quality, in a concept of ethics broader than the more traditional stress on duty, obligation and justice. In her research on moral development in young boys and girls, Gilligan showed that boys tended to resolve disputes by stressing rules and insisting on rights, while girls were more inclined to accommodate themselves to the needs of others and to the needs of maintaining friendly relationships. As a result, girls had a different approach to ethics, namely, a caring perspectice. In contrast, what Gilligan calls the justice framework of morality refers to those moral approaches that put a stress on what is obligatory or permissible for us to do in the light of principles. In this view, right action is action mandated or permitted by principles of various kinds. The two most notable principles cited in this context by contemporary philosophers are utility and the categorical imperative. The first enjoins us to do whatever leads to the greatest pleasure/happiness/preference-satisfaction for the greatest number, while the second enjoins us to do whatever we can consistently and universally want everyone to do. These two principles are each said to be overarching for the moral life and to explain the moral force of more specific principles such as those of benevolence, and of not lying, stealing or committing murder. Although the philosophical literature is full of debates between proponents of either principle, I want to take them together as exemplifying the justice perspective. Moreover, with its stress on law and duty, the natural law tradition should be included in this perspective.

The elucidation of the 'caring perspective' in ethics has encouraged proponents of the emotional concept of nurse caring to see such caring as morally excellent and as providing sufficient ethical justification for caring actions. For example, in a recent survey by Rita Manning, nurse caring was seen to constitute in itself a moral challenge to the objectified and bureaucratised organisation of much clinical practice (Manning 1998). This is because such caring is said to comprise moral attention, sympathetic understanding, relationship awareness, accommodation and response. All but the last of these are emotional and attitudinal stances that are assumed to give a positive moral quality to caring in the clinical context. In contrast, the justice perspective, with its stress on rights, principles and duties, would focus on the action that a nurse performs or fails to perform rather than on the motivations or feelings of that nurse. For this reason it aligns readily with what I have called the behavioural concept of caring in nursing. If all that matters ethically is the proper performance of professionally caring actions, then it will be principles and duties rather than feelings and motivations that are appealed to in evaluating the moral status of those actions. Moreover, the way we can be assured that an action is morally right in the justice perspective is by validating the reasons that prompted the agent to act. If those reasons were rationally consistent with the relevant principles, then the action would be right. The emotions or motivations that the agent may feel in relation to the action are not relevant.

In this way the dichotomy between the emotional concept and the behavioural concept of caring aligns with the distinction between the caring perspective and the justice perspective in ethics. If this is right, then an indirect way of mediating the dispute between the emotional concept and the behavioural concept of caring is to resolve the debate between the caring perspective and the justice perspective. There is literature in moral theory that seeks to do the latter, namely, the literature of virtue ethics.

In this chapter I will explore the suggestion that caring in nursing is a virtue. I will show that this way of seeing caring gives proper weight to the emotional aspects of caring but also places appropriate stress on the behavioural and rational aspects. I will then justify the claim that the virtue of caring is valuable in itself and does not need a justice or principle-based form of ethical thinking to justify it or to show that it is morally right. If those virtue ethicists are right who say that virtue ethics can stand on its own as an action guiding ethics, then the justice perspective (which insists that a principle-based, impartial, objective and universalisable form of thinking is required to supervise, as it were, the emotional promptings of caring) will lose its claim to being the only valid ethical stance. I will also argue against those theorists who say that the emotion of caring and sympathetic rapport with patients are necessary and sufficient conditions for morally good action on the part of nurses. Caring is not just emotional or motivational, nor is it only a form of acting. I will suggest that a virtue such as caring can be analysed as an orientation of the self towards the world in characteristic ways. It is a comportment or orientation of the whole of our internal life, whether emotional or rational, and of our intentional actions. I will argue that the virtue of caring is an ethical form of dynamic orientation towards the world and is especially appropriate for people who look after other people in one way or another: a virtue especially but not exclusively appropriate to the health care professions.

VIRTUE ETHICS

The philosophical literature on ethics makes a distinction between a concern for what we should *do* on the one hand and the way we should *be* on the other (Haber 1993). The first of these focuses attention on action and the principles or rules in the light of which an action can be said to be right or wrong. It can also focus attention on the goods that an action may achieve or promote and on whether these goods make the action right or wrong. Alternatively, it can direct attention on to the type of action that it is and on the moral status of such an action in the light of natural law. This is part of the justice

perspective. A focus on the way we should be, on the other hand, leads us to ask about whether an agent is a good person, has admirable character traits, feels appropriate emotions, has appropriate motivations, acts with integrity, or acts in a way that expresses a positive disposition. In short, a focus on how persons should be generates a discussion that has come to be known in the philosophical literature as 'virtue ethics' (Oakley 1996, Statman 1997).

The recently renewed interest in virtue ethics was inspired by the suggestion that, in some circumstances, a person who acts from principle would actually not be acting well. An example is a person who visits his friend in hospital (Stocker 1976). If he made this visit on the basis of duty, we would think that there was something lacking. In such a context, we consider that acting well would consist in visiting the friend out of friendly feelings. Similarly, we may suppose that nurses who look after patients efficiently and effectively, but do so purely because they feel it to be their duty to do so, would be lacking in some way. We would like caring to add to the moral quality of the activity through being part of its motivation.

In contrast, the more traditional approach of principle-based moral theory and the justice perspective (which undergirds most of bioethics) implies that there is a distinction between caring on the one hand and practical reason or ethical thinking on the other. According to this concept, applied recently to nurse caring by Helga Kuhse (1997), caring belongs to those of our faculties that prepare for action rather than to the action itself. For Kuhse, caring is appropriate when it gives rise to sensitive awareness of the suffering and needs of patients so that morally correct decisions can be made, but the focus of ethical appraisal or decision should be on the actions inspired by caring rather than on the caring itself. It is desirable that nurses should be caring individuals, and it may even be useful that they be so, but this is essentially a private, emotional and non-moral matter. What really matters is what nurses do. Impartial ethical thinking should be used to evaluate and decide on this. We could see why Kuhse would take this position if caring were essentially an emotion as the emotional concept suggests. Although the assumption has been contested (Oakley 1992), it is often thought that emotions are not amenable to moral evaluation or ethical control. Hence the emotions that nurses feel during their practice would be irrelevant to the moral status of their actions. Moreover, as Kuhse insists, such emotions are often disruptive of ethical thinking and action. This is where the concept of caring as a virtue can mediate the dispute. Many virtue ethicists will insist that virtue is not an emotion. Moreover, for such theorists, virtue thinking replaces ethics conceived of as an exercise of practical rationality that appeals exclusively to principles or rules.

Before proceeding to develop these points, however, I should point out that, by focusing on virtue ethics, I am actually speaking about a wider range of matters than are covered by the justice perspective of ethics. When we speak of actions being right or wrong we refer to a set of moral standards with a finite range of applicability. They include actions that honour or violate rights, or actions that honour or violate requirements of duty. Clearly this is a limited range of actions. One of the authors who revived contemporary interest in virtue ethics (Anscombe 1958) did so by suggesting that the standard moral terminology centred on such words as 'right' and 'wrong' was too abstract and 'thin' to be of much day-to-day applicability. It would be better to use 'thick' words that give more substance to the moral judgement that we are making: words like, 'courageous', 'considerate', 'just', 'generous', 'callous' or 'insensitive'. This use of specific virtue or vice terms enriches our moral discourse. Moreover, when we speak about virtue and the evaluation of persons or actions as virtuous, we embrace a much larger range of matters. A nurse may be cheerful at work and will be liked and admired on that account. This involves a positive evaluation, though not a moral one. Nurses may be efficient, courteous, punctual, neat, sensitive to the needs of patients, or any one of a range of positive features that we do not normally think of as explicitly moral matters, yet we consider

them admirable. We think of cheerfulness, efficiency, courtesy and neatness as virtues. It has also been argued that virtue is needed in other areas in which right or wrong are not at issue (Griffin 1998). Examples would be matters about which the justice perspective of ethics is largely silent, such as courtesy, respect, trust and caring for others. Without these interpersonal sensitivities the ethical life is arid. There are also intrapersonal qualities like integrity and authenticity; without these virtues the moral life is cold, harsh and meaningless. By itself, the justice perspective seems too shallow.

We can see this by reflecting on the term 'a good nurse'. If we were to spell out what it is to be a good nurse, would we use only moral terms? Would we spell this out only with reference to a nurse's universalisable and publicly justifiable duties? I suggest that such a description would contain terms that are descriptive of admirable traits, most of which will go well beyond what morality requires. If we disapprove of what a nurse has done, are we always saying that that nurse has done the morally wrong thing? Could it not be that the nurse has made a mistake or been careless? We may be saying that the nurse seems a bit surly today, or a bit sloppy or off-hand with a patient. In short, our disapproval does not always imply that we are referring to a moral issue (Komesaroff 1995). We will, however, be referring to standards of behaviour that we regard as virtues. Michael Slote has argued that the discourse of virtue is marked by praise of people that is based on attributing admirable traits of character or characteristic motivations to them as well as on admiring their characteristic behaviour and the way in which they do what they do (Slote 1992). What we mean when we criticise people in the discourse of virtue is that we find their behaviour and the character that it expresses to be deplorable. In this way when we speak of a 'good nurse' we are engaging in the discourse of virtue. In a similar way, when we describe a nurse as 'caring', we are making use of the concepts of virtue ethics.

ACCOUNTS OF CARING IN NURSING

What, then, is caring? The behavourist concept of nurse caring analyses it as looking after or providing for the needs of the other. Strict behaviourist psychologists eschew all reference to the internal states of persons and seek to describe human phenomena just in terms of what can be observed. Thus, a behaviourist account of caring would allude just to caring behaviours. Nurses would be said to be caring on this account if they evinced caring behaviours, where a 'caring behaviour' is defined as an activity that observably helps or meets the needs of someone else. Many would agree that such an analysis is inadequate if it is based solely on a description of behaviour rather than on an imputation about, or a reflective awareness of, the internal states of the agent.

It would be a slight improvement on such purely descriptive accounts to refer to nurses' 'dispositions' to caring behaviours. This would at least refer to the inner life of nurses in some way. A typical behaviourist will explicate a disposition by offering some counter-factual or subjunctive statements specifying what a person with the caring disposition would do if occasion demanded it. A typical example is given by Richard Brandt in his analysis of sympathy.

' … is sympathetic' would presumably include the following: (1) … would feel disturbed, other things being equal, if he perceived some sentient being to be in acute distress. (2) … would feel relieved, if he perceived a being in distress in process of being helped, provided he had earlier felt discomfort at the person's distress. (3) … would be motivated to relieve the distress, if he believed that he could do so and that no one else would if he did not. (4) … would feel guilty, other things being equal, if he perceived distress he thought he could relieve but did not, provided justifying or excusing considerations were absent. (5) … would notice a case of distress, if he were presented with it perceptually. (6) … would remember a previous case of distress, if he had noticed it before, and were now in a position to give relief (Brandt 1970, p. 29-30).

This account refers to a number of mental or psychological states of the person who is said to be sympathetic. In appropriate circumstances such a person would feel certain emotions, would be motivated to do certain things, would notice certain things, and would remember certain things. In a similar way, a caring nurse could be said on such a dispositional account to be one who would be motivated to help a patient if that patient were in need, or who would speak in a kindly manner to a patient if that patient were lonely or anxious, and so on. By specifying how the nurse would react in a range of typical circumstances, the behaviourist is giving an operational and observable account of what the disposition of caring is. Although this behaviourist account makes some reference to what is going on within the psychological make-up of the nurse, it is not, however, telling us what the motivational basis of these reactions is. It is not telling us what caring is as an internal, subjective and motivational comportment.

Caring in nursing is not just a set of psychological states or emotions that we can understand only insofar as they are manifested behaviourally or in emotional reactions. What caring produces in the way of sensitive perception, emotional reaction, or helpful behaviour is not the only indicator of what caring is. What I have characterised above as the emotional concept of caring is certainly more eloquent in giving us a richer and more subjective account of caring as a motivation and as an ideal quality of relationships with patients. However, the critics of this concept have made some valid points. First, the concept is often articulated in vague and florid terms. Secondly, caring in this sense is often irrelevant to the professional activities of nurses. When engaged in routine tasks, attending in operating theatres, or occupying other roles that do not permit interpersonal relationships, this concept of caring seems marginal. Thirdly, it is often impossible to care for 'difficult' patients in this emotional way. Lastly, sometimes the best way to do the job is with a minimum of emotional distraction; deep emotion can sometimes be unwanted and unhelpful.

The idea that caring is a virtue suggests an account that avoids both the dryness of the behaviourist concept and the sometimes romanticised rhetoric of the emotional concept. This account would go beyond mere dispositions or counterfactuals on the one hand, and emotional hyperbole on the other, in order to give a substantive account of the inner, psychological dimension of caring for the person who cares. In order to see what this account would be like, it will help to explore what Aristotle said about virtue.

ARISTOTLE ON VIRTUE

Aristotle began his analysis with the view that everything in the world, especially living things, had a specific *ergon* or tendency towards fulfilment (Aristotle 1941 trans); so a stone, when dropped from a height, had a tendency to fall towards the earth, a plant had a tendency to grow, animals had tendencies to forage, and so forth. The more complex an item was, the more such tendencies it would have, although these would combine together holistically to form the distinctive mode of being of that thing. Human beings were seen as highly complex beings with a large number of tendencies. However, the summation of these tendencies, the one ergon that summed them all up and marked out the distinctive character of human beings, was the tendency towards achieving *eudaimonia* or 'happiness'. Eudaimonia was both the goal of all human striving and the fulfilment of all human tendencies. A well-lived human life, therefore, was a life that fulfilled its tendencies and thereby achieved eudaimonia. A virtue was a trait of character that allowed us to achieve this goal and which, in its very exercise, would be the fulfilment of a tendency. Being virtuous was the fulfilment of the tendencies of being a human being and hence it created the happiness of the virtuous person. Happiness was not some sort of external reward at which the virtuous agent aimed. It was both the implicit internal goal and the effect of acting well.

There is no thought here about doing the right thing or acting morally. Aristotle did acknowledge that there were things that it would be wrong for anyone to do: things like adultery, theft, and murder, but he took it for granted that everyone understood this and that no one would be tempted to think that murdering someone could be any part of an answer to the question of how we should live our lives. What we would think of today as moral prohibitions of this kind were not up for discussion in Aristotle's text because attitudes towards them were not optional and were not a matter for individual judgement. For Aristotle, the issue was: How should we live well? not: What is the morally right thing to do?

However, it should not be thought that Aristotle's account of virtue in terms of the fulfilment of one's tendencies meant it would be virtuous for persons to do whatever they felt an inclination towards. Some thought should be given to what should be done in order to ensure that excesses or deficiencies of desire or emotion would be avoided, and in order to ensure that the action was appropriate to the situation at hand. Although he did not use the word 'right' in our modern sense of 'morally obligatory or permitted', he did think that we should apply standards to our own behaviour. As Aristotle put it:

Both fear and confidence and appetite and anger and pity and in general pleasure and pain may be felt both too much and too little, and in both cases not well; but to feel them at the right times, with reference to the right objects, towards the right people, with the right motive, and in the right way, is what is both intermediate and best, and this is characteristic of virtue (1106b17-23).

The key point here is that acting virtuously involves judgement. Because of this need for judgement about (non-moral) rightness, this account of virtue makes room for practical reason. Indeed, there is one virtue, the having of which implies having all the others, namely, the virtue of *phronesis*, which is usually translated as 'prudence' or 'practical wisdom' (see Ch 2). This virtue is a virtue of our thinking, but it also involves our desires and emotions because it includes the ability to perceive and to judge what is ethically important in a situation. It includes, in other words, caring and sensitive perception. Prudent persons are those who can appreciate the particular situations in which they find themselves, understand the means that they could use to achieve their goals, and be sensitive to which of their desires and which of the desires of others in that situation should be responded to and to what extent. The prudent person is the one who can consistently make judgements about the rightness or appropriateness of what is to be done and be motivated by these judgements to act in accordance with them. It is this centrality of judgement in virtue that allows the concept to combine the best of what both the emotional and the behavioural concepts of caring are trying to convey to us.

To explain this I want to highlight two important features of virtue in Aristotle's account: its dynamism and its holism. By its dynamism I refer to the suggestion that the very nature of human existence is to be a movement towards the goal of its own fulfilment. Human beings do not just react to things passively or follow rules mechanically in their behaviour. They do not just respond to stimuli. They seek after things and project their desires and aspirations upon the world so as to change it. They seek their own fulfilment. They are creative. It is the form given to this dynamism that is or is not virtuous. If this dynamism is structured by agents and by the surrounding society in such a way as to lead to the perfection of their faculties and to the constitution of their eudaimonia, then it is virtuous and the things that these persons characteristically do will be virtuous. It is this dynamism that captures the important emotional and motivational aspects of action that the caring perspective on ethics stresses.

The other point about Aristotle's account of virtue that should be highlighted is that it is holistic. Aristotle may be thought to be compartmentalising human existence by ascribing a number of distinct tendencies or functions, including desire and rational thought, to human beings. However, by suggesting that all these functions serve the single quest for eudaimonia, Aristotle ascribes a singleness of purpose to human life that combines all of the tendencies and functions together. Virtue consists in the functioning well of all the aspects of our being so as to constitute happiness. The well-

functioning of the whole person involves feeling rightly, as well as thinking rightly. The quest for perfection and eudaimonia will infuse and engage all of the activities and faculties of virtuous persons. Whether we are thinking of the emotions they feel, the attitudes that such persons have towards the world, the way they tackle practical problems, the kinds of friends that they enjoy being with, the activities that they will find satisfying and worth while to perform, the profession they take up, the ideals they subscribe to, or the kinds of ultimate hopes that they hold for the future, these elements will all be suffused by, and expressive of, their virtue. In everyday life, this virtue will come to expression in the way that they deliberate and decide about what to do. Aristotle does not distinguish sharply between desires and inclinations to act on the one hand and reasons for action on the other (Hursthouse 1997). The key point for us is that this holism embraces the important impartial and rational aspects of action that the justice perspective on ethics stresses.

There is one virtue that Aristotle specifically identifies as having this holistic scope, namely, that of prudence or *phronesis*. Such virtues as temperance, courage, generosity and wisdom come into play only in specific circumstances and on particular occasions, but a virtue like phronesis is relevant to all aspects of life and would ideally come to expression throughout it. Whenever a person judges a situation consistently with their comportment towards life and with reference to everything that is ethically important in it, and then acts in accordance with that judgement, that person is exercising phronesis.

CARING DEFINED

I want to suggest that caring can also be understood as a holistic virtue in this way. Rather than being, like courage, a trait that lies dormant and comes to expression only as specific occasions demand, it is a framework or a form given to all the aspects of our existence insofar as that existence expresses our caring for others. Although there is a concern for oneself involved in caring, as Nel Noddings reminds us (Noddings 1984), I want here to stress its directedness upon others. Accordingly, as I have argued in a previous publication:

caring [is] the comportment of the self towards others, which has the inherent goal of enhancing the existence of those others, whether they are others in intimate relation to me, others for whom I have professional responsibility, or others with whom I identify simply because they are compatriots, coreligionists, or fellow members of the human race (van Hooft 1999, p. 190) .

In speaking of an 'inherent goal' here, I mean that, as a caring person, my own existence achieves its fulfilment or perfection by virtue of the way I care for others. The fulfilment of my own tendencies is the implicit, inchoate and internal goal of my actions. Some of my actions will have the well-being of others as an explicit goal, and one that is conceived of as external to me. Nevertheless, if I am a caring person, that external goal will correspond to the fulfilment of my internal tendency. It is by virtue of this internal goal that my success at being a caring person will be partly constitutive of my eudaimonia. Caring in this sense is a virtue, and acting from this virtue will be acting well.

It has been argued (Bowden 1997) that caring is not the same virtue across various domains. It takes different forms in various contexts such as mothering, friendship, citizenship and nursing. I could add that it would be different again in such professional contexts as teaching or social work. Accordingly, I will have to add further specifications to the account of caring that I have just given if I want to apply the concept to health care professions such as nursing, medicine and the many other kinds of health therapy that are practised in the world today. I would suggest that, applied to the professions of health care, caring should be seen as a comportment towards others that has the inherent goal of enhancing the health-related existence of those others. The virtue of caring in nursing is an even more specific form of this virtue as applied to the professional nursing context. Accordingly, nurse caring will be the comportment of the nurse towards others, which has the inherent goal of enhancing the health-related existence of those others for whom the nurse has professional responsibility. In my definition of caring cited above I mention three alternative, but not mutually exclusive, bases for caring: intimacy, professional responsibility and identification or sympathy with others based on seeing them as in some respects like me. I would argue that nurse caring should be primarily based on professional responsibility (van Hooft 1987). Although intimacy and identification may occur in the context of professional health care, it is neither necessary nor in many cases desirable for the virtue of caring as it is evinced in nursing. Professional responsibility is a necessary and sufficient basis for this form of the virtue of caring.

In rejecting intimacy, sympathy and identification as necessary bases for nurse caring, I am rejecting some aspects of the emotional account of caring. However, I retain the central tenet: that nurse caring is a professional orientation of the nurse's whole being to the health-related well-being of patients. I also add the Aristotelian thought that this orientation includes sensitive and rational judgement leading to appropriate action. This thought allows a tempered version of the emotional concept to enrich the behavioural concept of caring with an account of the appropriate internal states of the caring nurse.

DOES ACTING VIRTUOUSLY REQUIRE EXTERNAL JUSTIFICATION?

It is an implication of this account of nurse caring as a virtue that actions which express this virtue do not require further rational justification in terms of moral principles in order to be deemed morally correct. However, not only Kuhse but also many other moral theorists would object to this implication (e.g. Griffin 1998, Sher 1998). Their view is based on the justice concept of morality that focuses upon the rightness of action. They say that virtue is merely instrumental towards acting rightly and that the justification of virtue arises only from the rightness of the act that it helps one to perform. Influenced by the modern concept of morality as being directed upon the issue of defining and doing what it is right to do, these philosophers say that, while virtues are useful in that they give us the skill, strength, habit or disposition to do the right thing, the important thing is to do what is right (where that is defined in terms of one or other moral principle). The virtues are useful or even essential in helping us to succeed in this. Such virtues as courage or persistence may help us to face the difficulties that stand in the way of doing the right thing. Such virtues as temperance and moderation may help us to overcome temptations that would lead us astray, and virtues such as sympathy and caring will help us to notice the features of a situation so that we can recognise what our obligations are. Again, virtues like benevolence and charity will be the habit or disposition to help others so that it is psychologically easier for us to do what is right. In these ways of thinking, doing what is right is still what is most important and is decided upon with impartial and rational thought, and virtues are seen as useful but inessential psychological tools, dispositions or strategies for acting in accordance with principle.

Applying the instrumental view of virtue to nursing, we could say that to be a virtuous or caring nurse is to have what it takes to work effectively and with commitment towards restoring or preserving the health of patients and members of the broader community. This idea will be open to considerable elaboration but the main point is that virtue is here being understood in instrumental terms. It would not be said from this point of view that virtue is its own fulfilment or is intrinsically valuable. Rather, it is valuable because it conduces to a good that is other than that virtue itself, namely, health or whatever other values may be considered to be the internal goods of the practice of nursing. If caring were seen as a virtue central to the profession of nursing, it would thus be understood in instrumental terms. Caring is good because it helps nurses to achieve their professional goals. Although these goals will be assumed in a day-to-day context, they can and should be discursively justifiable. However, such justification would, once again,

appeal to reason and, perhaps, to moral principles. As such, on this view, the virtue of caring is still secondary and subservient to the impartialist thinking of the justice perspective.

One interesting challenge to the view that virtues are valuable only insofar as they lead us to adhere to principles comes from Walter Schaller (1990). He argues against what he calls 'the standard thesis', which is that people can do their duty even when they do not have the relevant virtue, that the virtues are dispositions to obey moral rules, and that they therefore have only an instrumental value. He does this by showing that the duty of beneficence does not specify just what one is required to do in any given situation (just how much help is one obliged to give and how often?). Therefore it is best to have the virtue of benevolence. This virtue will lead one to judge what is needed and to act well in any given situation. Moreover, the concept of virtue will justify criticism of a person who fails to act well. A person cannot be criticised for failing to help in any given circumstance if the only requirement is a vague duty of beneficence, whereas we can criticise such a person for failing to be benevolent. Schaller also illustrates his point with reference to gratitude. The duty of showing gratitude cannot require only behaviour because such behaviour is meaningless unless the person actually feels gratitude and thus has the virtue of gratitude. It seems to me that this analysis applies also to caring. It is not enough to fulfil the duty of care by doing all that a caring practice requires; one must also feel it. Like gratitude and many cases of benevolence, one's actions do not actually convey the help unless they are felt as grateful, benevolent or caring by the recipient. Therefore the virtue is primary, and the action merely its expression. One cannot fulfil one's duty without first having the virtue. In these cases, like that of visiting one's sick friend, virtue is a necessary constituent of acting well.

To see why this is so, it is important to notice that Aristotle did not say that the virtues are useful to us in that they assist us in achieving eudaimonia. Rather, being virtuous constitutes that state of happiness, along with other felicities of life such as health and having good friends. It follows from this that virtue does not need an external justification. It is, as it were, its own reward. It will be an intrinsic good. Its justification will be internal in the sense that it is constituted by the fulfilment of the contextual goals of the agent. On this argument my proposal that virtue does not need any external justification from moral theories or principles would be established. The standard to be realised by virtuous action is set by what virtuous persons do, rather than by some universal criterion of goodness or justice.

However, there are commentators who say that the main problem with virtue ethics understood in this way is that it is circular. Virtue is said to be what the good person does and the good is said to be what the virtuous person aims for, so can the good be defined independently and transculturally? Although this is a larger question than can be dealt with in this chapter, I would want to follow the lead of Alasdair MacIntyre (1981) and suggest that this challenge need not force us back to mere subjectivism or individual preference as to what constitutes the good life and moral rightness. Specific forms of life do posit goals for human endeavour. We may think of specific communities or professions and point to goals that everyone in that community or profession shares or should share. Members of a religious community may share the goal of service to God, while members of the legal profession may share the goal of pursuing justice. In this way the profession of nursing may share the goal of restoring or preserving the health of patients and members of the broader community. Even though specifying the goals of a profession can be a fascinating and contentious exercise, as recent discussions within the profession of medicine show (Hastings Center 1996), the point that MacIntyre (1981) would make is that, if such non-universal goals that are internal to professions, cultures or 'practices' can be specified, then virtue can be defined as traits of character or as habits that are conducive to the attainment of those goals. As MacIntyre puts it: 'A virtue is an acquired human quality the possession and exercise of which tends to enable us to achieve those goods which are internal to practices and the lack of which effectively prevents us from achieving any such goods' (p. 178).

I ignore the instrumentalist tenor of this definition and cite it only to show that, within particular ways of life, communities and professions, one can specify goals, goods and ideals of character, which, even if they do not derive from universal goods, can be derived with sufficient objectivity from the agreed goals and goods internal to those ways of life and professions. Such goals and ideals are not just the preferences of the relevant people. They operate in the ethical lives of individuals as ideals with sufficient objectivity to constitute a challenge to their merely selfish desires. A community consensus is both necessary and possible for the grounding of the goods that define virtues (Slote 1992).

Martha Nussbaum has also made this point. Nussbaum (1998) argues against the claim that Aristotle's concept of virtue is relativist by showing that Aristotle's strategy is to mark out areas of moral concern that can reasonably be taken to be transcultural, and then to indicate what the proper (or 'mean') response to each should be. This appropriate response will be called a virtue. Although there may be local differences in how the latter are described, Aristotle would argue that some can be seen to be better than others by any rational being and that adherence to local tradition is not the final appeal. Reference to universal forms of human flourishing on his part makes that move easy, but even without this it is an empirical claim of Nussbaum's that there are indeed common concerns to human nature, and that there can be objectively resolvable debate about what responses to them are best. These concerns are: mortality, the body, pleasure and pain, cognitive capability, practical reason, early infant development, affiliation and humour. A good response to these is sought in differing cultural contexts and there is a remarkable congruence of cultural ideals relating to them. This points to a kind of pragmatic objectivity in defining what virtue is in each of these areas of concern.

If the virtue of caring provides an

appropriately objective standard for ethical action, then how is this standard put into effect? The sort of caring ethics that I would espouse makes virtuous character rather than right action the central issue (although actions can also be described as virtuous). From the perspective of an agent who is considering options in an ethically complex situation, there simply is no question of which of the options is right. I would say that there is something highly artificial and excessively impartial about anyone asking themselves that question. The question is: What should I do? This question concerns itself with the exigencies of the situation, with what the patient needs, or with how the family members of the patient feel, or with how they see the meaning of what is happening. It also concerns how nurses understand themselves as moral agents. Caring nurses will consider the particular and immediate circumstances of the situation and their own role in it. They will feel called upon to act by those circumstances. Sometimes they will feel called upon to act in contrary ways, so that they have to decide which action option to pursue. Even if they have to make explicit decisions of this kind, their consideration of the issues will be in 'thick' moral terms such as: What will relieve the most suffering? Or, How can I provide the most comfort? Or, What would it be fair to do? Or, What do the goals of my profession suggest here? It would be altogether too abstract and 'thin' to ask: What is the *right* thing to do?

It must be admitted that the questions: What would be consistent with my virtuous character to do? And, What is the caring thing to do? are equally artificial. Virtue ethics no more provides formulae for decision making than does principles-based ethics. In real life situations agents focus on the realities in front of them. What marks them off as virtuous in general or caring in particular is the way in which they focus upon these realities. To return to our earlier example, visiting a friend in hospital is virtuous when the way it is done is out of friendly feelings rather than as the result of a principled decision procedure. This does not mean that the friend will have asked himself what a virtuous character would do in such a situation. He simply feels that he is being consistent with his own self-image as a friend by doing it. He expresses his friendship by doing it. Doing it *that* way makes it a virtuous thing to do. Similarly, the caring of nurses does not ground a new kind of decision procedure; rather, it characterises the way that nursing is performed so as to make it virtuous.

CONCLUSION

The concept of caring in nursing, conceived of as a virtue, transcends the debates in moral theory between the caring perspective in ethics and the justice perspective. Just as a person who evinces phronesis feels rightly, thinks rightly, and thereby acts virtuously, so the caring person feels caringly, thinks caringly, and thereby acts virtuously. Caring conceived of in this way is neither merely an interpersonal emotion nor just a professional practice; it is the very ethical life of nursing.

REFERENCES

Allmark P 1995 Can there be an ethics of care? Journal of Medical Ethics 21 (1): 19-24

Anscombe G E M 1958 Modern moral philosophy. Philosophy: Journal of the Royal Institute of Philosophy 33 (124): 1-19

Aristotle. Nicomachean ethics. In: McKeon R trans 1941. The basic works of Aristotle. Random House, New York, p. 935-1126

Benner P, Wrubel J 1989 The primacy of caring: stress and coping in health and illness. Addison-Wesley, Menlo Park, CA

Blustein J 1991 Care and commitment: taking the personal point of view. Oxford University Press, New York

Bowden P 1997 Caring: gender-sensitive ethics. Routledge, London

Boykin A, Schoenhofer S 1993 Nursing as caring: a model for transforming practice. National League for Nursing, New York

Brandt R 1970 Traits of character: a conceptual analysis. American Philosophical Quarterly 7 (1): 23-37

Curzer H J 1993 Is care a virtue for health care professionals? Journal of Medicine and Philosophy 18 (1): 51-69

Fry S T 1989 The role of caring in a theory of nursing ethics. Hypatia 4 (2): 88-103

Gilligan C 1982 In a different voice: psychological theory and women's development. Harvard University Press, Cambridge MA

Griffin J 1998 Virtue ethics and environs. Social Philosophy and Policy 15 (1): 56-70

Haber J G (ed) 1993 Doing and being: selected readings in moral philosophy. Macmillan, New York

Hanford L 1994 Nursing and the concept of care: an appraisal of Noddings' theory. In: Hunt G (ed) Ethical Issues in Nursing. Routledge, London, p. 181-197

Hastings Center 1996 The goals of medicine: setting new priorities. An international project of the Hastings Center. Hastings Center Report 26 (6): S1-S27

Hursthouse R 1997 Virtue ethics and the emotions. In: Statman D (ed) Virtue ethics: a critical reader. Edinburgh University Press, Edinburgh, p. 99-117

Komesaroff P A 1995 From bioethics to microethics: ethical debate and clinical medicine. In: Komesaroff PA (ed) Troubled bodies: critical perspectives on postmodernism, medical ethics, and the body. Melbourne University Press, Melbourne, p. 62-86

Kuhse H 1997 Caring: nurses, women and ethics. Blackwell, Oxford

Leininger M M (ed) 1981 Caring: an essential human need. Slack, Thorofare, NJ

Leininger M M (ed) 1988 Care: the essence of nursing and health. (Human Care and Health Series). Wayne State University Press, Detroit

MacIntyre A 1981 After virtue: a study in moral theory. Duckworth, London

Manning R C 1998 A care approach. In: Kuhse H, Singer P (eds). A companion to bioethics. Blackwell, Oxford, p. 98-106

Nelson H L 1992 Against caring. Journal of Clinical Ethics 3 (1): 8-15

Noddings N 1984 Caring: a feminine approach to ethics and moral education. University of California Press, Los Angeles, CA

Nussbaum M 1998 Non-relative virtues: an Aristotelian approach. In: Sterba J P (ed). Ethics: the big questions. Blackwell, Oxford, p. 259-276

Oakley J 1992 Morality and the emotions. Routledge, London

Oakley J 1996 Varieties of virtue ethics. Ratio (New Series) IX (2): 128-153

Roach M S 1992 The aim of philosophical inquiry in nursing: unity or diversity of thought? In: Kikuchi J F, Simmons H (eds). Philosophical inquiry in nursing. Sage, Newbury Park, CA, p. 38-44

Roach M S (ed) 1997 Caring from the heart: the convergence of caring and spirituality. Paulist Press, Mahwah, NJ

Schaller W 1990 Are virtues no more than dispositions to obey moral rules? Philosophy 20 (Jul): 1-20

Sher G 1998 Ethics, character, and action. Social Philosophy and Policy 15 (1): 1-17

Slote M 1992 From morality to virtue. Oxford University Press, New York

Statman D 1997 Introduction to virtue ethics. In: Statman D (ed). Virtue ethics: a critical reader. Edinburgh University Press, Edinburgh, p. 1-41

Stocker M 1976 The schizophrenia of modern ethical theories. Journal of Philosophy LXXIII (Aug 12): 453-466

van Hooft S 1987 Caring and professional commitment. Australian Journal of Advanced Nursing 4 (4): 29-38

van Hooft S 1995 Caring: an essay in the philosophy of ethics. University Press of Colorado, Niwot, CO

van Hooft S 1999 Acting from the virtue of caring in nursing. Nursing Ethics 6 (3): 189-201

Wallis M C 1998 Responding to suffering: the experience of professional nurse caring in the coronary care unit. International Journal for Human Caring 2 (2): 35-44

Watson J 1985 Nursing: the philosophy and science of caring. Colorado Associated University Press, Boulder, CO

Watson J 1988 Nursing: human science and human care: a theory of nursing. National League for Nursing, New York

Wilkes L M, Wallis M C 1993 The five C's of caring: the lived experiences of students of nursing. Australian Journal of Advanced Nursing 11 (1): 19-25

2

Caritative caring ethics: a description reflected through the Aristotelian terms phronesis, techne and episteme

Maj-Britt Råholm

Caring is essentially a way of being alongside someone. In order to do this, we need first of all to be able to be deeply in touch with our own needs and values. Only in this way can we understand others. In this chapter, Maj-Britt Råholm leads readers to those deep and sacred aspects of life and living, where religious language needs to be used to convey what is meant. Concepts like 'communion' and 'bearing one another's burden' are considered and described in this chapter in the light of Aristotle's work, to lead to an understanding of what nursing is most essentially about.

INTRODUCTION

There is tension at the heart of modern health care. At a time when the ethics of health provision is constantly under scrutiny, too little attention is paid to 'care' as part of an ethical relationship and 'caring' as an expression of our humanity (Peacock and Nolan 2000). The International Council of Nurses *Code of Ethics for Nurses* (2000) states that 'Nurses have four fundamental responsibilities: to promote health, to prevent illness, to restore health and to alleviate suffering'. The Code further states that: 'The nurse carries personal responsibility and accountability for nursing practice and for maintaining competence by continual learning'. The American Nurses Association accepted a new version of its *Code of Ethics for Nurses with Interpretive Statements* in 2001 (American Nurses Association 2001). The first six statements focus on the individual ethical responsibilities of

nurses in clinical situations, and the primary focus of the first statement is on the ethical principle of respect for the inherent dignity of each person and the non-prejudicial care of all clients.

In Finland, a strong emphasis was placed on caring activities in nursing up to the Second World War (Tolonen 1995). The idea of caring and the attitudes necessary for caring were so often expressed that it must mean that they were considered to be of great importance for caring to take place. These ideas were largely forgotten by nurses after the Second World War, when ethics was more marked by thinking in terms of rules and results. Yet, even during periods when devotion to the calling, a spirit of service, humility and charity were replaced by efficiency, speed and knowledge, nurses looked for an ethics where love was a central concern (Tolonen 1995). The importance of character building and disposition for caring is also emphasised by Helena Leino-Kilpi (1990) and Unni Lindström (1992).

Current models of ethics education used in baccalaureate nursing programmes reflect a strong justice orientation to the neglect of the care dimension, despite the essential nature of care to the nursing profession (Crowley 1989). Although Lawrence Kohlberg (1981) viewed the ethics of justice as the primary ethical perspective, he admits that it needs to be supplemented by care. According to Carol Gilligan (1982), the moral problem arises from conflicting responsibilities rather than from competing rights, and requires for its resolution a mode of thinking that is contextual and narrative rather than formal and abstract. Per Nortvedt (1998) believes that an ethic of care in nursing has so far failed to present a thorough study and philosophical discussion of how emotions may give access to what is morally relevant in situations, and how they play a role in moral judgements. Nortvedt (1993) argues that care-based ethics is compatible with judgement based on universal impartial principles. However, an ethic of care articulates other important aspects of morality and moral behaviour than simply justice, although this is central to the main impartialist theories. Research to date in the field of nursing ethics has overlooked the nature of the guiding moral framework of nursing practice and has focused primarily on moral reasoning and moral behaviour among nurses (Cooper 1991).

Maritta Välimäki and co-authors (2000) provide an overview of all theses published on nursing ethics (n = 89) in Finnish universities between 1984 and 1997. There was no predominant research theme, but most of the work dealt with different aspects of nursing care, that is, the ethical principles of care. The authors point out that it will be important in future to clarify the theoretical points of departure of ethical research in relation to nursing and how these are to be applied in practice. Co-operation between the various caring science institutions in Finland, and also internationally, will be important in this respect.

According to Aristotle, reality (ontology) has a deep dynamic dimension. Exploring reality must also include a search for the basic (ethical) dynamic process of revealing (and being witness to) this knowledge in caring for the suffering human being. With ethics as the starting point, metaphysics will become meaningful (Lévinas 1988). Relying on Aristotle's (1967, 1976, 1987 trans) two different forms of knowledge—*phronesis*, which he himself also refers to as ethical competence, and *techne*—this chapter attempts to capture the distinctive features of the ethics of caring, where the deepest incentive to caring is love (Eriksson 1990, 1995, 2001, Lanara

1981, Roach 1992, Watson 1988). I will combine these two forms of knowledge in the field of caring science (*episteme*) and indicate how caritative caring ethics could find expression in education, research and practice.

THE SUFFERING HUMAN BEING

Caring ethics deals with the basic relationship between the suffering patient and the nurse. How the nurse meets the patient (a person who is ill or suffering) is an ethical act. The prevalence of encounters with suffering in nursing is emphasised by recognising that the Latin roots of the words 'suffer' and 'patient' are strikingly similar, both meaning 'to bear'. To be a patient, then, means to suffer, at least from the standpoint of etymology (Rodgers and Cowles 1997). Commonly identified elements of suffering are: distress, alienation and despair (Frankl 1986, Kleinman 1988, Travelbee 1971). According to Eric Cassell (1992), suffering occurs and is expressed not only physically, psychologically and socially, but also transcendentally. The importance of the loss of transcendence in suffering is suggested by how suffering may be overcome by transcendent means such as spirituality (God, purpose and meaning of life).

Most nursing school curricula address the pathological nature of illness, the nursing care of clients who are ill, the prevention of illness, and the promotion of health. There seems to be minimal discussion, however, both in nursing curricula and in textbooks, of the alleviation of suffering or of how nurses know that someone is suffering (Gunby 1996). Suffering can be studied only as human suffering; it constitutes a basic structure in a human being's understanding of his or her life situation. The deepest suffering can be likened to having been deprived of one's existential possibilities, being faced with an ontological crack that splits the whole existence of the patient (Lindström 1999). Nina Monsen (1990) sees human vulnerability in relation to one's dependence on the surrounding world. The struggle is thus an important inherent element in everyone, a prerequisite for becoming a whole human being. Suffering is the basic category that gives cause for caring and is the basis on which caring science knowledge develops. The struggle with suffering is a life-and-death struggle between good and evil, suffering and joy. In this struggle, in which a human being fights against evil and violation, there are, according to Katie Eriksson (1993, 1994) two possibilities: to fight and be reconciled, or to give up. To fight, and so to turn towards the wished-for and what is not yet, implies that one takes one more step towards death. Suffering is always a 'dying', even when it leads to new life, for suffering also implies growth. If no reconciliation can be achieved, there is a slow process of dying, where the manifestations of soul and spirit are often the first to fade away (Eriksson 1993).

Suffering is not a feeling, an experience or an abstract idea; it is ontological in character. Suffering becomes comprehensible only when it is related to a human being or is seen in a context. The movement of suffering occurs between two poles: by being confirmed by care-givers patients can experience suffering as meaningful, making it possible to realise their inmost beings. Compassion is more than just a natural response to suffering; rather, it is a moral choice (von Dietze and Orb 2000). If the ethical act does not take place, the patient may experience his or her suffering as unbearable and this prevents his or her movement in relation to the self and to others. Unbearable suffering is in its most intense form difficult to express explicitly, and the ethical act in caring implies, for instance, that the care-giver finds the concealed and hidden language together with the patient. The nurse can be with the suffering person in loving and ethically appropriate ways as the person finds new ways of becoming. The way out of isolated and mute suffering leads through expressing suffering together with a compassionate other that enables the sufferer to intercept the suffering and deal with it in the framework of narrative. That one should bear the burden of the other is the simple and clear call that comes from all suffering (Younger 1995).

The nurse and teacher Karin Neuman-Rahn

(Matilainen 2000) describes spiritual suffering as hard to interpret and as always subjectively experienced, and thus unique. We may even offend patients by underestimating their spiritual insight and intellect because of their spiritual suffering. According to Neuman-Rahn the depth of suffering can be judged only subjectively; no outsider can measure it.

When a patient expresses fear of dying or a sense of alienation from God, how easy it would be for the nurse to reply: 'Hold on to that comment and let me call the chaplain for you.' The only problem is that the patient, for whatever reason, has specifically chosen that nurse as someone safe to hear of his or her spiritual wrestling. This does not mean that the nurse takes the place of the chaplain, but rather recognises the invitation to enter this place of spiritual suffering. The invitation is to come alongside and be allowed to see, to share, to touch, and to hear the brokenness, vulnerability and suffering of another (Pettigrew 1990).

In her study, Susan Gunby (1996) confirmed that nursing students can learn how to care for those who are suffering by utilising the four patterns of knowing delineated by Barbara Carper (1978). The students revealed that individuals who are suffering often need someone to help, understand, be with them, be truly present, and exhibit genuine compassion for them. It is possible to experience the suffering of others by entering into their world through their metaphors and the language by which they express their suffering, and their movement beyond it.

Nel Noddings (1984) argues that we should not put strict ethical principles before an ethic of caring for the person experiencing suffering in a concrete lived moment. Caring means a stir of emotion, a call to the heart rather than the mind.

DIGNITY

The first concept, in my opinion, that is inherent in phronesis (i.e. ethical competence) is human dignity. When studying the history of nursing, one becomes aware of how nurses have always had to struggle in order to maintain the dignity of human beings and to uphold their absolute values. In this struggle, nurses have sometimes submitted to the reductionist paradigm with its mechanical way of looking at human beings, while fighting for the values that make caring an act of love and compassion. The deepest ethical motive in all caring is to show respect for a human being's absolute human dignity (Eriksson 1990, 1995). Jean Watson (1988) points out that we must show consideration and dignity in relation to ourselves before we can respect and care for others with consideration and dignity. In caring, the sympathetic human qualities of a caregiver may be reflected in the patient. Caring may well begin as an ideal but has to be translated into a will, an intention and a deliberate judgement that is demonstrated in concrete acts. The act of caring must be focused on the protection, enhancement and preservation of human dignity (Watson 1988).

In her study, Mary Solveig Fagermoen (1997) addressed the research question: What are the values underlying nurses' professional identity? The results showed that human dignity and altruism were the most prominent moral values of nurses. According to Anna Söderberg and co-authors (1997), dignity opens the registered nurses to the ethical dimension and this, in turn, counteracts the risk of dehumanising care in technocratic environments (here the context of intensive care). Richard Dworkin (1995) argues that dignity is a fundamental and universally necessary condition for worthwhile human life and that a human being's critical interests are sacred. Gadow (1988) describes a patient who was seriously burned many years ago: 'As long as the patient and his nurses remained mutually engaged in each other's vulnerability and its alleviation, the existential distance between them diminished' (p. 13-14). In her ethical model based upon the covenant of care, the crucial distinction is not that between health and death, but that of alleviating versus intensifying vulnerability. Confirming the patient's absolute dignity here means a mode of responding to the other's plight that exceeds an epistemological determination and becomes an ethical involvement. The possibility of shaping one's life

oneself is intimately connected with one's human dignity. This dignity is lacking when the care-giver is caring only for the body (giving medication and doing various caring routines). In this situation one is forced to deny an archetypal inner need that is painful later to recover because it brings back to life one's deep longing for love and closeness (Lindström 1994).

Irene von Post's (1999) study shows that, when natural care is excluded from professional care, the dignity of the patient is violated. Sigridur Halldórsdóttir (1996) mentions three important components that are inherent in professional caring: competence, caring and connection. The basis of her theory is that there is a difference between caring and professional caring. From the data it can be concluded that competence administered with compassion is an essential component of professional caring. These three aspects also have consequences for our fundamental attitudes, values and inherent ethical readiness to address the patient and to confirm the patient's dignity as a human being. Being professional also involves being human, that is, being open to experiences that make it possible to step aside and let the other come forward. It is the facial expressions that, according to Peter Kemp (1991), penetrate one's living space and appeal in a way that no sensuous entity can. It is this appeal that matters for the care-giver at the bedside. Listening and whole-hearted presence are the prerequisites for receiving the message. It is the other's appeal for love and communion that makes the care-giver responsible at that moment. A human being's vitality and his or her courage to face life are deeply rooted in past experience of dignity, that person's own holiness and dignity.

THE RESPONSIBILITY

The second important concept inherent in phronesis is the idea of responsibility, the idea of which helps us to interpret and meet the innermost desires of suffering patients by being truly present (Råholm and Lindholm 1999). According to Nel Noddings (1995), 'oughtness' is part of our 'isness' (p. 187–188) and this is the root of our responsibility to one another. In many common human situations we respond spontaneously to another's plight. This spontaneous response she calls 'natural' caring. In contrast, ethical caring does have to be summoned. The 'I ought' presents itself, but encounters conflict. On these occasions we need not turn to a principle; more effectively, we turn to our memories of caring and being cared for, and a picture or ideal of ourselves as care-givers.

As a nurse, I have to respond to the cared-for who addresses me in a special way and asks me for something concrete and, perhaps, even unique. The motive to care arises on its own; it does not have to be summoned. Ethical responsibility arises when the other person is met face to face (Lévinas 1988). Emmanual Lévinas describes this face as the ethical resistance to encroachments on human rights, a non-physical resistance to all forms of outrage. Lévinas (1993) later speaks about the vulnerability to the other's look as fundamental in ethics. It is by virtue of my own vulnerability that I become an individual taking responsibility for the other person's welfare. Lévinas' contribution can be said to consist in counteracting the reduction to invisibility of the unreduceable remnant of suffering, which, in his opinion makes us endlessly responsible. This responsibility can even become vicarious for the other, that is, an abandonment of one's self to the other (G Torrkulla, unpublished work, 2001). Responsibility can be divided into outward and inward. Outward responsibility consists of the rules and duties of the profession, but inward responsibility is more than a 'feeling' or 'moral obligation': it is 'engrossment', in Noddings' (1984) words. This requires of nurses the capacity to see what the other sees and feel what the other feels.

Entering into 'communion' is, according to Lévinas (1988), to create possibilities for the other. He points out that seeing the other as one's son implies establishing something 'beyond the possible'. It means being able to get out of the confinement of one's own identity and what belongs to one. It is fatherhood, one of the profoundest forms of communion. Lévinas

emphasises our human vulnerability, which is characteristic of us as ethical individuals. Jaspers (1963), on the other hand, sees the other as indispensable because of the help he or she can give us in order to cope in borderline situations (Kemp 2001).

In order to describe the nature of responsibility in the caring communion, one can start from an interpretation of the face from the point of view of three different dimensions. First of all, the face may mean that we meet fellow human beings, not only persons with a diagnosis. Life is to be understood as a relation between a subject that is directed towards something, and an object, towards which the subject is directed. The other is also a subject, so communication may be a battle between faces that attempt to objectify the other. In this way nurses may prove their superiority over the other or else they are themselves objectified by the other and cast down their eyes with shame. Secondly, the other's face does not merely see or look at something, but appeals. Thirdly, the face may simply confirm our existence. The face does not only express a demand but indicates also how we should respond to the demand and thus confirm each other's existence (P Kemp, unpublished work, 2000).

According to Knud Ejler Løgstrup (1994), trust is an inherent element in every meeting between human beings. The other person is entrusted to us and it is in our power to accept or reject that person. The other person expects love from us; his or her trust claims our attention. This demand is silent, and silence implies that it becomes a part of us, independent of our own attitude. The patient's words thus convey the ethical message and the acceptance of this ethical act lies in the appeal. According to Nortvedt (1998) one can choose not to respond to a patient's discomfort; it may even be morally appropriate to do so, owing to other patients' salient needs, but one cannot choose the fact that, when seeing the other's need and expectation, that responsibility has already come to the forefront, that vulnerability has become one's affair. Judgement is secondary. Responsibility becomes more prominent than knowledge, or to put it in Lévinas' words, 'being-for precedes being-with' (1988, p. 113). The care-giver's responsibility lies in the challenge of being able, in a certain light, to mould this profoundly ethical demand and act accordingly. Thus the ethical scene in its nakedness and its immediacy appeals to the care-giver. The scene can be a meeting with a patient with severe chest pain in a hospital corridor who is experiencing deep sorrow, or a coronary artery bypass patient who has just been extubated in an intensive care unit and experiences fear and insecurity. It is because of the face that we shut out each other from, or invite each other to, our innermost selves.

Illness becomes a language that indirectly reveals how patients view themselves and life. Therefore the symptoms become a face that reveals the whole. Illness allows a patient to open what is normally concealed. Care-givers have a face of their own: that of their professional role. What do they want patients to see in this face (Brager and Wisløff 1990)?

Responsibility can be likened to the ethical scene. To confront a patient's pain is also to experience his or her suffering, and, surely, to encounter a person's suffering is to encounter something moral. To be touched by a patient's suffering is to encounter responsibility. To be sensitive to a person's human experiences is the sine qua non of moral responsibility.

THE CARITAS MOTIVE

The third important concept inherent in phronesis that constitutes the foundation in caritative caring ethics is the caritas motive. Western traditions of caring up until the eighteenth century were founded primarily on Christian principles. The patient, whether physically or mentally ill, was taken to a safe place or sanctuary that provided escape, respite and care. In these sanctuaries, the sick were nurtured both physically and spiritually by carers whose remit was to provide non-judgemental companionship. By recapturing the human aspects of caring we move care away from a position where patients are seen as 'cases'

and subjected to judgements and therapies, towards an ethical relationship (Peacock and Nolan 2000). A concept that has a long history can retain its original meaning or content and at the same time acquire a great many connotations in the course of time. In pre-Christian times, 'love' was considered to be the highest principle governing human behaviour. In his *Ethics* (1976 trans) Aristotle defines the highest form of love (Philein) as the desire for another person's good for that person's sake. On the other hand, Aristotle acknowledges that we can love other persons in an objectifying manner, not for 'their own sake' but only in relation to ourselves. With the rise of Christianity, love was redefined according to the New Testament Agape. Caritas is the Latin translation of the Greek word *agape*, which means divine and unselfish, spontaneous love. In caring contexts, caritas should be a motive for action (empathy and compassion), a principle of action (namely, the principle of equality), and an ethical ideal, conforming to the saying, 'do to others what you would have them do to you' (Matthew 7:12). This ethical ideal does not have a settled core. It receives its definite content in the meeting between fellow human beings in the caring reality (Barbosa da Silva 1999). According to Søren Kierkegaard:

Indeed the life of love is recognisable by its fruits, which make it manifest, but the life itself is still more than the single fruit and more than all the fruits which one could enumerate at any moment. Therefore the last, the most blessed, the absolutely convincing evidence of love remains: love itself, which is known and recognized by the love in another (Kierkegaard 1962, p. 33).

There is an ancient idea that the eye of the mind sees concepts, and the eye of the heart sees by entering into a caring relationship (Roach 1998). Being there in a true caring communion with the patient means letting love flow rather than doing something ethical. It is the nurses' answer to the innermost desire of the patient, which is sometimes unspoken, for the deepest suffering has no voice. It is not enough to be there; it is in the way, the 'spirit', in which it is done that the caritative ethic in care becomes important, with the idea of love as the leading motive (Eriksson 1995). An ontology of caring provides both a starting point and a context for reflections about ethics and the ethical life. Truth is known not from a set of facts, but rather by being authentic, choosing beauty, and sharing the experience of unconditional love. The core of ethics means that one has an obligation to love. An ontology of caring as the sacred art of love is the awareness of love and givenness because there is love, a force that is the basis of all intersubjective experience. Caritative caring ethics means also that we are willing to paint and repaint constantly our self-portrait in caring for the suffering human being (Råholm and Lindholm 1999).

THE ART OF CARING

In my view, the concept of the art of caring is inherent in Aristotle's second form of knowledge, techne. We sometimes speak as if caring did not require knowledge, as if caring for someone were simply a matter of good intentions or warm regard (Mayeroff 1971). The caring relationship is the existential condition. A human being is open and vulnerable in a caring relationship and can be received or rejected. Receiving the patient is an ethical demand that has no place in utilitarian ethics (Noddings 1984). Caritative caring completes advanced technological and scientific knowledge. Through the ages, caring has involved a combination of 'hand', 'head' and 'heart', or, in other words, caring has been art, technology and science. By implementing the caritas motive, caring achieves its profoundest form and appears as ethical throughout (Eriksson 1990, 1995, 1997). In ethics there are theories concerned with disposition, situation and virtue, which have been used as explicit frames of interpretation in caring ethical research connections (Eriksson 2001). According to Annatjie Botes (2000), the two different perspectives, the ethic of justice and the ethic of care, represent opposite poles. The ethic of justice constitutes an ethical perspective in terms of which ethical decisions are made on the basis of universal principles and rules, and in an impartial and verifiable manner with a view to

ensuring the fair and equitable treatment of all people. The ethic of care, on the other hand, constitutes an ethical approach in terms of which involvement, harmonious relations and the needs of others play an important part in ethical decision making in each situation. This could be compared with what Mary Silva and colleagues (1995) describe as the ontological and epistemological dimensions of ethical knowledge. The ontological dimension is the ethical being, that is, what one ought to be morally, and entails certain traits that are valued in nursing, such as empathy and compassion. The epistemological dimension, on the other hand, deals with the scope, kind, trustworthiness and justification of ethical knowledge, or the moral validity of what one must do. Carper (1978) identified ethical knowing as one of the fundamental patterns of knowing in nursing. This pattern is essential to nursing because the discipline has a moral obligation to provide service to society and is responsible for conserving life, alleviating suffering and promoting health.

According to Carper, one of the 'patterns of knowing' central to caring is that of 'aesthetics: the art of nursing' (Carper 1978, p. 16). In ancient Latin and Greek the relevant terms (*ars* and *techne*) referred generally to any skilled activity. The dialogue that occurs in the meeting between care-giver and patient means that the care-giver is present at the moment when the patient turns to her or him. This immediate presence is a way of being that can be neither planned beforehand nor described in technical terms. According to Otto Bollnow (1976), the encounter between the caregiver and the patient could be described as an existential (life-changing) situation where the care-giver touches the very essence of the patient's life and makes him or her grow. It is the nurse's sincerity and genuineness (making use of the entire self) as essential to the transpersonal relationship, theorised that such relationships include an important metaphysical component, which is realised in the 'presence of the union of two persons' souls' (Watson 1988, p. 70–71). One can have an exact objective knowledge of another human being, of that person's psychological type and his or her foreseeable reactions, but nevertheless be ignorant of that human being's essential ego and self-knowledge. Only by identifying oneself with someone else's personal entity, by making an existential penetration into the core of that person's being, will it be possible to get to know that person in his or her existing reality (Tillich 1977). These words comprise a profound ethical message, that is, one's own existence becomes part of somebody else's existence.

In Lévinas' vision the individual is not a 'case' to be measured, documented and quantified, but an 'infinity'. The face-to-face encounter is at the heart of the caring relationship. All too often patients complain that they have not been 'heard' by their doctor, nurse or carer (Forrest 1989). John Peacock and Peter Nolan (2000) argue for urgent re-examination of what we understand by 'care'. At a time when the ethics of health provision is constantly under scrutiny, too little attention is paid to 'care' as part of an ethical relationship and 'caring' as an expression of our humanity.

Confirming the other means touching that person in a profound sense, and the question is whether it is even possible to touch another human being without being touched oneself. The very act of turning to another human being is creative, and the humble sounding-board of the care-giver is a prerequisite for confirmation to take place (Lindström 1994).

In a study by Dagfinn Nåden (1999), invitation and confirmation were two important themes that emerged from conversations with patients. The results also showed that despondency and exposure occurred when this confirmation was not forthcoming. Although these concepts were implicit in the statements of the care-givers, they were not explicitly expressed. The art of caring could be portrayed, as Milton Mayeroff (1971) states, by showing my commitment to the other; holding myself out as someone who can be depended on. If there is an acute break in this relationship because of my indifference or neglect, I feel guilty, as if the other were to say, 'Where were you when I needed you?' This guilt results from my sense of

having betrayed the other, and my conscience calls me back to it. The more important this particular other is to me, the more pronounced is my guilt. The story of the Good Samaritan describes the very essence of the art of caring. The Samaritan does not respond to the situation in a detached way, as if indifferent to the suffering of the other person, but becomes engaged in the reality of the injured and bleeding traveller. The traveller is cared for by the 'deeply moved' Samaritan, who attends to his physical wounds and pain at the roadside, but who also takes him into the protection of a nearby inn (McAllister and Ryan 1996). According to Anthony Tuckett (1998), caring becomes identifiable as an act that is inclusive of a compassionate and empathetic 'way of being', and which strives to protect the other because of deep concern for that other's threatened personhood. The nurse, in ministering to a dying man whose only home is a bus shelter, but who is living the most sacred and solemn moment of his life's journey, is responding as a human person. Although the nurse's professional role imposes a duty, intentionally chosen, when she or he decided to become a nurse, there is a sense that caring is fulfilling a human need within the nurse. Not to care is somehow to lose one's being; in caring, the nurse becomes a more authentic human being (Roach 1997).

CONCLUSION

In this chapter I have tried to capture the most central elements in caritative caring ethics, starting from the Aristotelian division of various forms of knowledge: phronesis and techne. Without having previously made use of the concept, we can now see that the old Aristotelian phronesis knowledge has formed the basis for the learning and practice of good actions, and is also visible in the care-giver's approach. Phronesis is a form of knowledge that has its theoretical foundation in ethics. It emphasises deliberation and moral action and, according to Don Flaming (2001), should replace the phrase 'research-based practice' as the guiding light for nursing practice. When Aristotle wrote about techne, he was thinking of art and craft, or handicraft. An artist starts working with devotion and care but is nevertheless open to the unforeseeable in the artistic process. When we speak about the ethics of care, as carers we must reflect on what we are bringing to the caring dynamic: is it the rigour of mathematical certainty, or values that are growth producing (Devlin 1996)?

What emerges in the art of caring is the suffering human being, that person's dignity, the care-giver's ethical responsibility, and the love of one's neighbour. These form at the same time important building blocks in the caring science development of knowledge (episteme) and in the subdiscipline of caring ethics. Epistemic knowledge is considered as true knowledge and deals with the necessary knowledge. Theory is the form of activity that is performed by the epistemic human being and describes, reflects and analyses the caring situation. The caritas motive then constitutes the value basis of caring science (episteme) and the ethical reason for all caring. In the widest sense this also includes caring administration and caring didactics. In Lévinas' (1988) opinion, an ontology that is not subordinated to ethics is impossible, because the understanding of 'being' in general cannot indicate and control the genuine relationship with another person, but it is this relationship that must determine the understanding of being. Nursing knowledge (epistemology), and its essence in being-for-the-other (its ontology), means being responsible for the other, being answerable for the other's condition, pain and vulnerability (Nortvedt 1998).

The web of meaning connected with caring (i.e. what unites and ties together and confers meaning on caring) is made up of the caring communion. True communion implies that one has come out of oneself and entered a relationship in which one is prepared to create possibilities for the other. The basic prerequisite for such communion is to be found in the caritas motive, which constitutes the fundamental value and the ethos that makes communion an ethical act.

The task of basic research in caring science is to raise new questions concerning caring ethics. The main function in clinical caring science is to create an ethical model for caring where the clinical reality with all its patterns and nuances is reflected through the core of caring science. In theoretical scientific discussion, more thought should be devoted to how research on questions concerning the ethics of caring can lead to new discoveries and development in the formation of the theory and what consequences this will have for the care-giver in a clinical context. The challenge lies in the ability to implement this theoretical knowledge about caritative caring ethics in our everyday practice. More clinical nursing research is needed, especially at Master's degree level, in order to get more nurses involved in answering questions concerning the fundamental patterns of an ethic of care.

In this way phronesis, techne and episteme will reach their perfection in the meeting with suffering patients.

REFERENCES

American Nurses Association 2001 Code of ethics for nurses with interpretive statements. ANA, Washington DC

Aristotle Den nikomachiska etiken (The Nicomachean ethics). (Ringbom M trans 1967). Holger Schildts Förlag, Helsingfors (in Swedish)

Aristotle Ethics. (Thompson J A K trans 1976). Penguin, Harmondsworth

Aristotle Om själen (The soul). (Gabrielsson J trans 1987). Daidalos, Göteborg (in Swedish)

Barbosa da Silva A 1999 The concept of caritas. Ylihoitajalehti 27 (4): 4–8

Bollnow O F 1976 Eksistensfilosofi og pedagogikk. (Philosophy of existence and pedagogy). Christian Eilers Forlag, Copenhagen (in Danish)

Botes A 2000 A comparison between the ethics of justice and the ethics of care. Journal of Advanced Nursing 32 (5): 1071–1075

Brager E, Wisløff D S 1990 Så länge vi lever (As long as we live). Cappelens Forlag, Oslo (in Norwegian)

Carper BA 1978 Fundamental patterns of knowing in nursing. Advances in Nursing Science 1 (1): 13–23

Cassell E 1992 The nature of suffering: physical,

psychological, social and spiritual aspects. In: Starck P, McGovern J (eds). The hidden dimensions of illness: human suffering. National League for Nursing Press, New York, p. 1–11

Cooper M C 1991 Principle-oriented ethics and the ethics of care: a creative tension. Advances in Nursing Science 14 (2): 22–31

Crowley M A 1989 Feminist pedagogy: nurturing the ethical ideal. Advances in Nursing Science 11 (3): 53–61

Devlin B 1996 Ethics and the spirituality of caring. In: Farmer E (ed). Exploring the spiritual dimension of care. Mark Allen Publishing, Dinton, p. 52–60

Dworkin R 1995 Life's dominion. Harper Collins, London

Eriksson K 1990 Mot en caritativ vårdetik (Caritative caring). (Report from the Department of Caring Science, no. 2/1990.) Åbo Akademi, Vasa (in Swedish)

Eriksson K 1993 Moten med lidanden (Encountering suffering). (Report from the Department of Caring Science, no. 4/1993.) Åbo Akademi, Vasa (in Swedish)

Eriksson K 1994 Den lidande människan (The suffering human being). Liber Utbildning, Arlov (in Swedish)

Eriksson K 1995 Mot en caritativ vårdetik (Towards a caritative caring ethics). (Report from the Department of Caring Science, no. 5/1995.) Åbo Akademi, Vasa (in Swedish)

Eriksson K 1997 Perustutkimus ja käsiteanalyysi (Basic research and concept analysis). In: Paunonen M, Vehviläinen-Julkunen K (eds) Hoitotieteen tutkimusmetodiikka. Werner Soderstrom Osakeyhtio Oy, Juva, p. 50–76 (in Finnish)

Eriksson K 2001 Vårdvetenskap som en akademisk disciplin (Caring science as an academic discipline). (Report from the Department of Caring Science, no. 7/2001.) Åbo Akademi, Vasa (in Swedish)

Fagermoen M S 1997 Professional identity: values embedded in meaningful nursing practice. Journal of Advanced Nursing 25 (3): 434–441

Flaming D 2001 Using phronesis instead of 'research-based practice' as the guiding light for nursing practice. Nursing Philosophy 2 (3): 251–258

Forrest D 1989 The experience of caring. Journal of Advanced Nursing 14 (10): 815–823

Frankl V 1986 Livet måste ha mening (Man's search for meaning). Natur och Kultur, Stockholm (in Swedish)

Gadow S A 1988 Covenant without cure: letting go and holding on in chronic illness. In: Watson J, Ray MA (eds) The ethics of care and the ethics of cure: synthesis in chronicity. National League for Nursing, New York, p. 5–14

Gilligan C 1982 In a different voice: psychological theory and women's development. Harvard University Press, Cambridge, MA

Gunby S S 1996 The lived experience of nursing students in caring for suffering individuals. Holistic Nursing Practice 10 (3): 63–73

Halldórsdóttir S 1996 Caring and uncaring encounters in nursing and health care – developing a theory [thesis]. Linköping University, Linkoping

International Council of Nurses 2000 Code of ethics for nurses. ICN, Geneva

Jaspers K 1963 Introduktion till filosofin. (Byttner A trans) (First published 1953 Einführung in die Philosophie (Introduction to philosophy). Piper, München.) Bonniers, Stockholm (in Swedish)

Kemp P 2001 Principper for omsorg (Principles of care). In:

Bjerrum M, Lund Christiansen K (eds) Filosofi. Etik. Videnskapsteori (Philosophy. Ethics. Theory of science). Copenhagen: Nørhaven Books, p. 179–184 (in Danish)

Kemp P 1991 Det oersättliga – en teknologietik (The irreplaceable – an ethics of technology). Brutus Östlings Bokförlag Symposium, Stockholm (in Swedish)

Kierkegaard S 1962 Works of love. Harper and Row, New York

Kleinman A 1988 Shame: the power of caring. Schenkman, Cambridge, MA

Kohlberg L C 1981 Essays on moral development. Harper and Row, San Francisco, CA

Lanara V 1981 Heroism as a nursing value. Sisterhood Evniki, Athens

Leino-Kilpi H 1990 Good nursing care. On what basis? [thesis] University of Turku, Turku (in Finnish)

Lévinas E 1988 Etik och oändlighet (Ethics and infinity). Symposium Bokförlag and Tryckeri, Stockholm (in Swedish)

Lévinas E 1993 Den annens humanisme (The humanism of the other). Aschehoug Forlag, Oslo (in Norwegian)

Lindström U 1992 De psykiatriska sjukskötarnas yrkesparadigm (The professional paradigm of the qualified psychiatric nurse) [thesis] Åbo Akademi, Vasa (in Swedish)

Lindström U 1994 Psykiatrisk vårdlära (Psychiatric nursing). Liber Utbildning, Uddevalla (in Swedish)

Lindström U 1999 Det psykiatriska vårdområdet – en deldisciplin inom vårdvetenskapen (Psychiatric care: a discipline within caring science). In: Janhonen S, Lepola I, Nikkonen M, Toljamo M (eds) Professori Maija Hentisen juhlakirja (Approaching the new millennium in caring science in Finland – dedication to Professor Maija Hentinen). Oulu University, Oulu, p. 65–72 (in Finnish)

Løgstrup K E 1994 Det etiska kravet (The ethical demand). Bokförlaget Daidalos, Göteborg (in Danish)

McAllister M, Ryan M 1996 The Good Samaritan: a revitalised narrative for nursing. Australian Journal of Holistic Nursing 3 (1): 12–17

Matilainen D 2000 Idémönster i Karin Neuman-Rahns livsgärning och författarskap – en idéhistorisk- biografisk studie i psykiatrisk vård i Finland under 1900-talets första hälft (Patterns of ideas in Karin Neuman-Rahn's life-work and writings – a study of psychiatric care in Finland in the earlier part of the twentieth century, based on biography and the history of ideas.) [thesis] Åbo Akademi, Vasa (in Swedish)

Matthew 7:12 The Holy Bible, New International Version 1986. Hodder and Stoughton, London, p. 883

Mayeroff M 1971 On caring. Harper and Row, New York

Monsen N K 1990 Det kjempende menneske (The struggling human being). Cappelens Forlag, Oslo (in Norwegian)

Nåden D 1999 Når sykepleie er kunstutøvelse. En undersøkelse av noen nødvendige forutsetninger for sykepleie som kunst (When nursing becomes an art) [thesis]. Åbo Akademi, Vasa (in Swedish)

Noddings N 1984 Caring: a feminine approach to ethics and moral education. University of California Press, Berkley, CA

Noddings N 1995 Philosophy of education. Westview Press, Boulder, CO

Nortvedt P 1993 Emotions, care and particularity. Vård i Norden, Nursing Science and Research in the Nordic Countries 13 (1), 18–24

Nortvedt P 1998 Sensitive judgement: an inquiry into the foundations of nursing ethics. Nursing Ethics 5 (5): 385–392

Peacock J W, Nolan P W 2000 Care under threat in the modern world. Journal of Advanced Nursing 32 (5): 1066–1070

Pettigrew J 1990 Intensive nursing care. The ministry of presence. Critical Care Nursing Clinics of North America 2 (3): 503–508

Råholm M-B, Lindholm L 1999 Being in the world of the suffering patient: a challenge to nursing ethics. Nursing Ethics 6 (6): 528–539

Roach M S 1992 The human act of caring. Canadian Hospital Association, Ottawa

Roach M S 1997 The convergence of caring and spirituality. In: Roach M S (ed) Caring from the heart. Paulist Press, New York

Roach M S 1998 Caring ontology: ethics and the call of suffering. International Journal for Human Caring 2 (2): 30–34

Rodgers B L, Cowles K V 1997 A conceptual foundation for human suffering in nursing care and research. Journal of Advanced Nursing 25 (5): 1048–1053

Silva M C, Sorrell J M, Sorrell C D 1995 From Carper's patterns of knowing to ways of being: an ontological philosophical shift in nursing. Advances in Nursing Science 18 (10): 1–13

Söderberg A, Gilje F, Norberg A 1997 Dignity in situations of ethical difficulty in intensive care. Intensive and Critical Care Nursing 13 (3): 135–144

Tillich P 1977 The courage to be (Modet att vara till). (Ahlberg A trans) Studentlitteratur, Lund

Tolonen L 1995 Etik och etikett i patientvården (Ethics and etiquette in nursing) [thesis]. Åbo Akademi, Vasa (in Swedish)

Travelbee J 1971 Interpersonal aspects of nursing, 2nd edn. Davis, Philadelphia, PA

Tuckett AG 1998 An ethic of the fitting: a conceptual framework for nursing practice. Nursing Inquiry 5 (4): 220–227

Välimäki M, Leino-Kilpi H, Tepponen H, et al 2000 Research on nursing ethics: an overview of academic theses in Finland 1984–1997. Hoitotiede 5 (12): 227–234

von Dietze E, Orb A 2000 Compassionate care: a moral dimension of nursing. Nursing Inquiry 7 (3): 166–174

von Post I 1999 Professionell naturlig vård ur anestesi- och operationssjuksköterskors perspektiv (Professional nursing care from the nurse anaesthetists' and operating room nurses' view) [thesis]. Åbo Akademi, Vasa (in Swedish)

Watson J 1988 Nursing: human science and human care. A theory of nursing. National League for Nursing, New York

Younger J B 1995 The alienation of the sufferer. Advances in Nursing Science 17 (4): 53–72

3

Virtue, nursing and the moral domain of practice

P. Anne Scott

To mention the word 'virtue' 20 years ago would have made nurses squirm. Anne Scott is one of the nurses who has helped to bring virtue ethics firmly into the arena of nursing and ethics, and today virtue ethics is one of the important approaches used. In this chapter, she details the origins of the theory and relates the theory to practice. What makes the practice of nursing special, and what makes a nurse act caringly, have been debated at great length. This may be looking in the wrong direction. By starting, as the ancient Greeks did, with the question of how we are to live well, we find that we have to answer in a different way. That way takes us to aspects of living and acting together and what that entails in terms of character and virtue.

INTRODUCTION

It is commonplace now in both literature and rhetoric to suggest that nursing is a moral practice or enterprise, or that it has a significant moral element. Nursing has been described variously as: a caring profession (Benner and Wrubel 1989), moral action (Atkinson 1997), containing a significant moral dimension (Griffin 1980, Sarvimäki 1995, Scott 1996), having a moral goal (Scott 1995) and as being a moral practice or enterprise (Nordvedt 1998). Bernadette Dierckx de Casterlé et al (1998) suggest:

Nursing practice primarily concerns the personal relationship between the nurse and the patient. This personal encounter calls for nurses to be responsible for the person for whom they are caring: meeting this 'otherness' incites nurses to transcend their

nursing routine and to find a personal response to the patient's problems. This requires nurses to undertake a critical and permanent reflection on their practice and on its whole context … This emphasis on the patient's well-being turns care into an ethical endeavour and requires moral maturity of the nurse (p. 832).

Per Nortvedt (1998) suggests that 'the essence of nursing knowledge and nursing performance cannot be understood merely as ontology (i.e. being-with-the-other). Nursing is basically being-for-the-other; it is responsibility; it is ethics' (p. 385).

Rather than getting swept away in the rhetoric, I think we need to pause and ask: What is being claimed of nursing here? We need to do this in order to begin to address the question: What is the relationship between nursing and the moral domain? It seems that there are two types of claim appearing in the literature. The strong claim is that nursing is a moral enterprise or practice. The weaker claim is that nursing contains a significant moral element. Thus, even if one is unhappy with the notion that nursing is a moral enterprise or practice, one may wish to argue that, nonetheless, nursing contains within its practice a significant moral element.

In order to examine the strong claim made above, one needs to ask what would count as a moral enterprise or what kind of practice would be considered a moral practice. It seems that there are a number of considerations, not the least significant of which is: What is meant by 'moral' here? We are aware that moral action and judgement is that which has to do with one's interactions with others. Ethics (the term is used interchangeably with moral here) Ian Thompson and co-authors (1994) tell us, is to do with the rights and wrongs of human behaviour.

Nurses constantly interact with others, with patients, clients, colleagues and so forth. It does seem to be the case that many nursing actions affect people, mainly patients. Do all nursing actions do this? Clearly this is not so. Filing, shifting beds, and numerous administrative tasks fall within the remit of nursing actions (i.e. actions regularly carried out by nurses). These actions cannot incontrovertibly be said to affect people.

Nonetheless one needs to ask how useful is this notion of an action that undeniably affects another person (people), as descriptive of the moral? Shopkeepers of all descriptions, in selling merchandise to customers, directly affect their customers. However, we do not normally consider shop-keeping as a moral enterprise. This seems to be a label that is reserved for activities like nursing, medicine and education. Why is this? What, if anything, distinguishes the person who goes into a boutique seeking help and advice on the purchase of a new suit, from the person who presents to an accident and emergency department seeking treatment and advice regarding an injury or accident?

Perhaps the needed distinction is between interacting with people and affecting them in a manner that directly benefits or harms them as people.

We have already seen that not all nursing activities do in fact have a direct impact on a person for good or bad. Thus it does seem to be the case that it would be very difficult to support the strong claim that nursing is a moral enterprise or practice, if by this is meant a practice whose entire activities fall within the moral realm. Furthermore, to try to do so could trivialise and thus undermine the importance of the moral dimension in nursing practice and those activities that do clearly fall within its area of concern. If not all nursing activities are moral activities, perhaps the practice of nursing is still a moral practice because it is entirely rooted in moral concerns.

Is nursing then a practice rooted in moral concerns? It may be useful to consider the motivation to become a nurse, the duties and obligations of the role, and the goal or aim of nursing practice. Regarding the motivation to nurse, this seems quite mixed: nursing has traditionally been an acceptable female profession; many enter nursing seeking a socially respected job and the possibility of continuous employment. There are also motivations that stem directly from idealism and a wish to be of service. There is also, in some societies, a status issue. The duties and obligations of the nursing role are largely socially determined and supported through licence to practice. Some of these duties are moral duties but some do not seem to have salient moral content, for example, the payment of the regulatory body's registration fee at the appointed time. I think the jury is out on the notion that nursing is entirely rooted in moral concerns, although there are a number of authors who claim this of both nursing and medicine. Thus I do not want to support the strong claim that nursing is a moral enterprise or a moral practice as such. However, it does seem perfectly possible to support the weaker claim that nursing has a significant moral element, indeed perhaps even a moral goal. This is the case for a number of reasons.

In the first place it is clear that some nursing activities do have a direct impact on a person or patient. That impact is to the benefit or detriment of that person. For example, careless or incompetent care can lead to injury, pressure sore development, lack of recognition of significant postoperative complications (BBC 1 Scotland 1999), or malnutrition (e.g. when staff do not ensure that debilitated, dependent patients can physically access their meals, once delivered to their trays).

We also know of many counter examples, such as that described by Anne Oakley (1993), of the young nurse whom the patient perceives as having a profound impact on his or her care. This may be the nurse who sits and listens, sensitively and intelligently, to a patient's concerns and then provides the needed information and support.

In the second place, the activity of nursing is directed towards an aim. I would argue that this aim or goal, patient comfort or wellbeing, is clearly a moral aim or goal because it has the essential element of some notion of the good for a person or patient as a human being. For example Steven Edwards (1998) describes the end of nursing as 'to promote health or well-being' (p. 399). This notion of the good for a human being and of the duty of nurses to promote this type of end is commonly discussed in our ethics literature, for example Martha Levine (1977), Sally Gadow (1980), Elsie and Bertram Bandman (1995), and Vangie Bergum (1994). It is also clearly iterated in the *Code of Professional Conduct* (NMC 2002). One can take this literature and the Code as one wants. Nonetheless it seems to me very hard to argue against the notion that the role of nurse or doctor primarily exists, and is sanctioned by society, to do people good. This good is not in terms of increasing their financial status or their attractiveness to the job market, but to do people good through caring for their health, and thus to do people good as human beings.

CURRENT THOUGHT REGARDING THE MORAL DOMAIN OF PRACTICE

Over the last 20 years or so, as interest in the ethics of health care and health care practice has gained momentum, the focus of attention from both academics and practitioners has tended to be on the notion and nature of moral duties. This is undoubtedly, and in no small measure, due to such influential publications as Tom Beauchamp and James Childress's *Principles of Biomedical Ethics* (1989) and the popularity of Kantian ethics in mainstream Anglo-American moral philosophy. However, a number of contributors to the health care ethics literature have, for a number of years now, tried to argue that within the health care and nursing context a virtue theory approach is needed at least as a supplement to this duty- and principle-based approach (Allmark 1998, Pellegrino and Thomasma 1993, Scott 1996).

WHY A VIRTUE THEORY APPROACH?

In the health care literature it is possible to identify clearly a concern that is focused on the person of the practitioner and on the abilities of the practitioner to interact in a humane, sensitive, compassionate and imaginative way with the human being who is that practitioner's patient (Toon 1993). Such elements as compassion, sensitivity and imaginative ability are dispositions or traits of the person's character, rather than duties of the role of health care practitioners. In discussing dispositions of a person's character, dispositions that are moral in nature, Aristotelian virtue theory provides a very useful framework.

It is possible that with further work the character traits of health care practitioners identified in the literature can be related to and supported by a theory of virtues. This is a position already evident in work such as Edmund Pellegrino and David Thomasma (1993). Such a perspective would help to broaden and enhance the approaches of duties, rights and consequences, which, until recently, predominated in bioethics. These latter principle-based perspectives tend to focus descriptions of the moral on rightness or wrongness of action, and to begin with the assumption that what matters is to have the correct beliefs about ethical questions. However, the ancient Greeks had another way of looking at these issues: '... the ancient Greeks started with a totally different sort of question; ethics is supposed to answer, for each of us, the question "How am I to live well?" .... "How should/ought/must I live in order to live the best life/flourish/be successful?' (Hursthouse 1987, p. 221-222).

Ancient Greek thought is the foundation of virtue theory and many philosophers agree that the theory is found in its most developed early form in the works of Aristotle (Foot 1978, von Wright 1963). An account of Aristotle's theory of the virtues is beyond the scope of this chapter. However, key sources remain Aristotle's *The Eudemian Ethics* (1992 trans) and *The Nicomachean Ethics* (1953 trans). It is generally agreed that the latter text is the more developed and inclusive version. The revised translation of *The Nicomachean Ethics* by John Ackrill and James Urmson (1980) contains translators' notes and commentary likely to be particularly useful.

According to Aristotle, and many developmental theorists since, moral development begins in childhood; Aristotle emphasises the vital importance of upbringing. It may be argued that this is really not very useful to educators in the health professions because our students are aged at least 17 years, and are generally considered to have been 'brought up' by this age. This perception (at one level obviously accurate) is presumably why many teachers of health care ethics say, with Steven Miles and colleagues (1989), that their function is not one of creating sound moral character or virtuous practitioners. However, there is at least an element of this perception that is, I think, mistaken. If one reviews the extensive literature on the process of professionalisation and its implications (Melia 1987), and gives credence to the recognised dehumanisation that takes place among medical and nursing students and personnel, then it becomes difficult to argue cogently that educational attempts in the opposite direction must necessarily be completely futile. Juxtaposing these factors alongside developing evidence of the impact that the culture and organisation of health care services has on our ability to perceive moral issues makes this a particularly pertinent discussion (Holm 1997). The important point here is that, if a practitioner does not recognise the moral, there is a danger that it will be coped with only accidentally, if at all.

Aristotle speaks of people's upbringing as being influential in their moral development. In terms of the practitioners of health care, it seems there should be overt (as well as the already apparent covert) recognition that there is a period of 'upbringing' in the professions, which, in terms of the moral behaviour of the practitioner, may be of similar importance as the influence of childhood upbringing is to the moral behaviour of the adolescent and adult. This notion suggests that it is important to provide student practitioners with appropriate role models, and to take seriously the Aristotelian idea of the importance of developing the habits appropriate to the virtuous person by observation of virtue in action. In Pellegrino's words: 'We have freely asserted that we are humane, and that students should also be, without providing consistent examples of this humanness in our attitudes and actions. This big gap, then, is an existential and behavioural one which curricular design alone cannot possibly close' (Pellegrino 1979, p. 205).

Developing the habits of the virtuous, from appropriate exposure and training, ultimately leads to the development of virtue in the individual. In virtue theory there is a difference between the person whose intentions are good and the good or virtuous person. The perceptions, emotions and desires of the latter are trained to see the reality of a situation as accurately as possible. The virtuous person is therefore more likely to be in a better position to be able to decide the direction within which good lies than is the person whose good intentions may spring from subconsciously selfish motives, or from a less than accurate perception of the situation.

According to Aristotle, virtues are states or traits of character. The right state of character is that state from which on each occasion the appropriate actions and emotions result.

The virtue of a thing is relative to its proper work. Now there are three things in the soul which control action and truth - sensation, reason and desire ... of these sensation originates no action ... what affirmation and negation are in thinking, pursuit and avoidance are in desire: so that since moral virtue is a state of character concerned with choice and choice is deliberate desire, therefore, both the reasoning must be true and the desire right, if the choice is to be good, and the latter must pursue just what the former asserts.

... The origin of the action - its efficient, not its final cause - is choice, and that total choice is desire and reasoning with a view to an end. This is why choice cannot exist either without reason and intellect or without a moral state; for good action and its opposite cannot exist without a combination of intellect and character (Aristotle 1980 rev trans, p. 138-139).

There are a number of points to note in the above excerpt. Perhaps the first is the importance given to choice in moral virtue. Actions involve choices. I choose to give the relevant information or I choose to withhold it. I choose to tell a lie or to tell the truth, and so on. However, Aristotle states that virtue does not involve only action, it involves appropriate emotion. It does not seem immediately evident how I choose my emotions. Most of us are familiar with the experience of: 'I wish I could stop getting so angry with X.'

VIRTUE AND EMOTION

Aryeh Kosman (1980) gives a detailed and lucid explanation of Aristotle's account of the virtues as complex states or traits of character, comprised of appropriate feelings and actions:

The doctrine of passive potentiality enables Aristotle to envision a state of character by virtue of which an individual has the power to be affected in certain ways, the capacity to undergo certain passions and avoid others. A moral virtue with respect to feelings or emotions is just such a capacity; it is the power to have and to avoid certain emotions, the ability to discriminate in what one feels ... A person may act in certain ways that are characteristically and naturally associated with a certain range of feelings, and through those actions acquire the virtue that is the disposition for having the feeling directly. Acts are chosen, virtues and feelings follow in their wake, though in logically different ways ... One does not have direct control over one's feelings, and in this sense the feelings are not chosen; but one does have control over the actions that establish the dispositions ... which are the source of our feelings .

... The question of moral choice in the deepest sense finally concerns questions of creating the conditions in which our actions and our feelings may be as we would wish them (p. 107–115).

This notion that our feelings follow our actions may on the surface seem rather convoluted. However, when one reviews theories related to attitude change and immersion desensitisation approaches to the treatment of phobias and trauma (Saigh et al 1996), one can argue that Aristotle's notion, that certain behavioural habits could lead to appropriate emotions, finds support in contemporary psychological theory.

A second point to note is the notion that how one feels about something is important, or has moral significance. On reflection this seems reasonable in terms of the character of the person. To help a colleague out of fellow-feeling is surely better than to help because one knows the boss is watching. Aristotle says that appropriate emotion is important from a moral point of view because without appropriate emotion virtue does not exist. Although accepting the Aristotelian position here, I would also want to claim that, in the health care context, appropriate emotion is not only morally very relevant, it is also essential to good practice. Without the appropriate emotional element, the practitioner cannot practice well. If one's emotion is not in tune with what one is doing then one is likely to be led astray; one's judgement may be affected by inaccurate perceptions and desires (Scott 2000).

THE IMPORTANCE OF VISION AND PERCEPTION IN VIRTUE THEORY

It is at this point that the importance of the notions of vision and perception enter virtue theory. As Myles Burnyeat (1980) points out: 'The noble and the just do not, in Aristotle's view, admit of neat formulations in rules or traditional precepts. It takes an educated perception, a capacity going beyond the applications of general rules, to tell what is required for the practice of virtue in specific circumstances' (p. 72).

The next question must be: What is educated perception and how does one get it?

The late Iris Murdoch (1970), in her essay, 'The idea of perfection', may provide some parts of the answer that we seek, when she says that 'where virtue is concerned we often apprehend more than we clearly understand and grow by looking' (p. 31). We come to see by attending properly, that is, completely and selflessly, to that at which we are looking. Murdoch (1970) borrows the notion of attention from the works of Simone Weil to express 'the idea of a patient, loving regard directed upon a person, a thing, a situation' (p. 40).

Perception is trained by practice; for example, a

learner driver will frequently misperceive potential sources of danger. Common misperceptions of this nature are speed and the distance away of other vehicles. This can lead to a learner driver entering a road without waiting for oncoming vehicles to pass because the learner mistakenly thinks that the other vehicles are sufficiently far away or moving sufficiently slowly to allow safe entry into another road. It is only with practice and experience that the driver's perception of actual and potential dangers become more accurate. In terms of virtue, emotion and perception are connected. The emotions one has about a situation, behaviour or event can influence one's ability accurately to perceive the situation. For example, if one is very angry at one's spouse for failing to be home on time as promised, the anger may prevent one from allowing one's spouse to explain what happened or from hearing any explanation given. This leads to an inaccurate perception of the actual situation that exists between one's spouse and oneself. If I have strong feelings of revulsion towards the act of abortion, this is likely to diminish seriously my ability to perceive accurately the situation of a young girl who concludes that the least bad decision she can make, in her particular circumstances, is a decision in favour of abortion. A training of the emotions is therefore important in achieving accurate perception.

Perfect virtue is unlikely to be found, except rarely (if at all), among human beings; but by practising virtue one comes to see more clearly the direction in which one should go and what counts as being worth while. It is said that the Inuit perceive at least 15 different shades of the colour white, their perception being developed and shaped by their environment. In a similar way, being educated by the practice of appropriate habits and attentive looking, helps one to achieve virtuous action and virtuous character, as well as to see what is most worth while and good to do.

Noble moral virtues ... are then, not simply dispositions to act in certain ways. They are more like skills which suit us for life generally - and still more like traits of character which not only suit us for life but shape our vision of life helping to determine not only who we are but what world we see (Meilaender 1984, p. 11).

ARISTOTELIAN VIRTUE THEORY IN HEALTH CARE ETHICS

As I suggested at the beginning of this chapter, there are concerns among both academics and practitioners that duty-based theories do not provide a sufficiently comprehensive framework on their own, within which to deal with the moral dimension of health care practice. Aristotle's virtue approach, based as it is on practical reason, is of value in supplementing the duty-based approach to health care ethics. This is the case for a number of reasons, among which is the general idea that people do not get on very well without virtues. As theorists such as Philippa Foot (1978) and Peter Geach (1977) have pointed out, the virtues are beneficial to human interaction and communication, and to the functioning of human society. This is surely at least as relevant to persons interacting in the health care context as it is to the wider society.

The idea that being good is important, and that to be good one must look at and work on one's character, has a deeply intuitive appeal. It also seems to be in tune with those in health care practice (and indeed among the recipients of health care) who suggest that the character of the practitioner is important and that this should receive at least as much attention in health care ethics as considerations of duty and rights.

Within the context of health care practice:

1. The right thing to do cannot always be laid down in a rule. Perception of the particular case or situation is needed.
2. It matters what one feels and thinks, as well as what one does.
3. Good and inspirational practice involves an element of perfection.

Within virtue theory, Aristotle makes similar claims. For example, he asserts that virtue concerns *perfection* of the human being in living a good human life.

How do these claims relate to health care and nursing practice?

It is not always obvious what one should do in a particular situation, or what one's duty actually is. Aristotle maintains that developing virtue will help us to see wherein the good lies. Appropriate example/exposure is elemental in virtue development. This forms the potential basis for good habit formation and education of the emotions and perception.

Appropriate emotion and accurate perception are, according to Aristotle, necessary elements for virtue to exist; therefore, appropriate emotion and accurate perception are important to morality. I want to argue that they are not only important to morality, they are also important to good health care practice. This is because, without accurate perception, the practitioner's judgement is constantly in danger of being misguided and faulty. Judgements regarding patients' needs, diagnoses and treatments are the bases of health care practice. If these judgements are in constant danger of being faulty, then practice itself rests on a very insecure foundation. Consistently good practice must have a secure foundation. Therefore the judgements on which practice rests must be as faultless as is humanly possible. Such judgements demand, among other things, appropriate emotion and accurate perception on the part of the practitioner.

This calls for the development of certain virtues in the practitioner, which in Aristotle's terms is a call to perfection. That is, practitioners are being called to find their *ergon* in the context of health care practice. This ergon is achieved by developing certain virtues. Thus practitioners will come to know and do the right thing, in the right way, for the right reasons, at the right time.

CONCLUSION

Much of the small amount of literature within nursing that focuses on a virtue approach has emphasised the character of the individual practitioner. This is almost certainly appropriate. However, there is a grave danger for nursing as a profession if this focus on the individual is to the exclusion of all other considerations. The individual practitioner does not exist in a vacuum.

Studies by Bowman (1995) and Holm (1997) provide crucial insights into the impact of organisational structures and culture on individual perception and moral sensitivity. To ignore such influences would perpetuate 'the sins of the code of practice', which place the entire responsibility for standards of care, and the human good that nursing can or should produce, exclusively on the shoulders of individual practitioners. Notions of shared or collective responsibility are thus completely ignored.

I wish to support the weak claim that nursing practice contains a significant moral element and a moral goal. To analyse this moral domain and best equip practitioners for a recognition of it in their clinical practice, virtue theory has much to offer. However there are also dangers for both patient care and our profession if we naively work from a superficial grasp of Aristotelian theory. One of these dangers is further to burden the individual practitioner and ignore our collective professional responsibility to ensure that the context of clinical practice is conducive to good patient care.

REFERENCES

Allmark P 1998 Is caring a virtue? Journal of Advanced Nursing 28 (3): 466–472

Aristotle The Nicomachean ethics (Ross D trans 1953, Ackrill J L, Urmson J O 1980 rev) (World Classics Series) Oxford University Press, Oxford

Aristotle The Eudemian ethics, books I, II, VIII, 2nd edn. (Woods M 1992 trans). Clarendon Press, Oxford

Atkinson J 1997 A descriptive and evaluative study of district nursing intervention with single homeless men from a private hostel in Glasgow [thesis]. Glasgow Caledonian University, Glasgow

Bandman E L, Bandeman B 1995 Nursing ethics through the life span, 3rd edn. Prentice Hall, Englewood Cliffs, NJ

BBC 1 Scotland 1999 Panorama, Monday 30 Sept 1999. 22.00–22.40 h

Beauchamp T L, Childress J F 1989 Principles of biomedical ethics, 3rd edn. Oxford University Press, New York

Bergum V 1994 Knowledge for ethical care. Nursing Ethics 1 (2): 71–79

Benner P, Wrubel J 1989 The primacy of caring: stress and coping in health and illness. Addison-Wesley, Menlo Park, CA

Bowman M 1995 The professional nurse. Chapman and Hall, London

Burnyeat M F 1980 Aristotle on learning to be good. In: Rorty A O (ed) Essays on Aristotle. University of California

Press, Berkley, CA, p. 69–92

Dierckx de Casterlé B, Roelens A, Gastmans C 1998 An adjusted version of Kohlberg's moral theory: discussion of its validity for research in nursing ethics. Journal of Advanced Nursing 27 (4): 829–835

Edwards S 1998 The art of nursing. Nursing Ethics 5 (50): 393–400

Foot P 1978 Virtues and vices. Basil Blackwell, Oxford

Gadow S 1980 Existential advocacy: philosophical foundation of nursing. In: Spicker S, Gadow S (eds) Nursing: images and ideals. Opening dialogue with the humanities. Springer, New York, p. 79–102

Geach P 1977 The virtues: the Stanton lectures (1973–74). Cambridge University Press, Cambridge

Griffin A P 1980 A philosophical analysis of caring in nursing. Journal of Advanced Nursing 8 (2): 289–294

Holm S 1997 Ethical problems in clinical practice. Manchester University Press, Manchester

Hursthouse R 1987 Beginning lives. Basil Blackwell, Oxford

Kosman L A 1980 Being properly affected: virtue and feeling in Aristotle's ethics. In: Rorty A O (ed) Essays on Aristotle. University of California Press, Berkley, CA, p. 103–116

Levine M E 1977 Nursing ethics and the ethical nurse. American Journal of Nursing 77 (5): 845–849

Meilaender G C 1984 The theory and practice of virtue. University of Notre Dame Press, Notra Dame, IN

Melia K M 1987 Learning and working: the occupational socialisation of nurses. Tavistock, London

Miles S H, Lane L W, Bickel J, Walker R M, Cassel C 1989 Medical education: coming of age. Academic medicine 64 (12): 705–714

Murdoch I 1970 Sovereignty of good. Routledge and Kegan Paul, London, p. 1–45

Nortvedt P 1998 Sensitive judgement: an inquiry into the foundations of nursing ethics. Nursing Ethics 5 (5): 385–392

Nursing and Midwifery Council 2002 Code of professional conduct. NMC, London

Oakley A 1993 Essays on women, medicine and health. Edinburgh University Press, Edinburgh

Pellegrino E D 1979 Humanism and the physician. University of Tennessee Press, Knockville, TN

Pellegrino E D, Thomasma D C 1993 The virtues in medical practice. Oxford University Press, New York

Saigh P A, Yule P A, Inamdar S C 1996 Imaginal flooding of traumatised children and adolescents. Journal of School Psychology 34 (2): 163–183

Sarvimäki A 1995 Knowledge in interactive practice disciplines [thesis]. Stockholm University College of Health Sciences, Stockholm

Scott P A 1995 Role, role enactment and the health care practitioner. Journal of Advanced Nursing 22 (2): 323–328

Scott P A 1996 Ethics, education and nursing practice. Nursing Ethics 3 (1): 53–63

Scott P A 2000 Emotion, moral perception, and nursing practice. Nursing Philosophy 1 (2): 123–133

Thompson I E, Melia K M, Boyd K M 1994 Nursing ethics, 3rd edn. Churchill Livingstone, Edinburgh

Toon P D 1993 After bioethics and towards virtue. Journal of Medical Ethics 19 (1): 17–18

von Wright S V 1963 The varieties of goodness. Routledge and Kegan Paul, London

4

Feminist ethics

Joan Liaschenko   Elizabeth Peter

Feminine ethics or feminist ethics? To make the distinction—and the point about each—Joan Liaschenko and Elizabeth Peter make a wide sweep of the background and history of ethics. Thus this chapter supplies some of the context that other chapters might have taken for granted. Their careful argument to reach their position as feminist ethicists is worth a careful read because it necessarily highlights the many areas of concern to all nurses. Aspects of political action, as described here, are not often heard or considered so clearly within nursing, but they need to be used more if nursing is to have a future at all.

INTRODUCTION

Our task in this chapter is to describe what is known as feminist ethics. This is not a small task, given that feminist ethics is not one but rather a range of approaches that challenge traditional ethics primarily in the two areas of virtue or character and cultural ethos. In sociological terms these domains are akin to the individual and the social world between which there is an inherent tension. One can look at the feminist challenges to these domains as an 'ethic of care' and an 'ethic of power' respectively (Tong, 1997). This chapter explores feminist ethics by examining the tension between these two ethics. We begin by describing the ways in which feminist ethics, as a general category, augments traditional ethics. The second part describes how feminist ethics, with its elements of care and power, is related to Lee Yearley's (1990)

articulation of the moral domains of injunctions, virtues and ways of life. In doing so, feminists also reveal the inherent tensions in these domains. In the third part we look at how nursing ethics scholarship has taken up care, power and feminist ethics in its endeavour to articulate an ethic for nursing that is not only coherent, but is sensitive to the complexities of moral life in nursing.

What makes feminist ethics feminist is the study of moral theorising with respect to gender. A feminist approach is defined by taking as its starting point the experience of women, by acknowledging that this experience is characterised by oppression and domination, and by its open commitment to changing the practices of this oppression and domination (Bell 1993, Brennan 1999, Browning Cole and Coultrap-McQuin 1992, Card 1991, Lengermann and Niebrugge-Brantley 1988, Purdy 1989, Tong 1997, Young 1990). Oppression refers to 'the institutional constraint on self-development' and domination refers to 'the institutional constraint on self-determination' (Young 1990, p. 37). Women are oppressed and dominated because they are women, not for reasons having to do with a particular woman. It is important that the vehicles for this oppression and subordination are institutional, which is to say the origins do not lie in any particular man but in a social system that privileges male interests. In her historical novel, *The Red Tent*, Anita Diamant (1997) tells the story from the Hebrew Bible of the Tribe of Joseph from the perspective of selected women. The individual male characters are depicted as both caring and abusive, but also revealed are the institutional forces extending beyond any individual man that shows that women are clearly property. The denial of women's right to vote until relatively recently in modern democracies is a contemporary example of an institutional constraint against women. The institutional aspect is crucial to understanding the feminist position.

There is, however, no single, non-disputed version of moral theorising that constitutes feminist ethics. This is not surprising, given that feminist theory is characterised by a multiplicity of perspectives in politics, epistemology, ontology and ethics (Tong 1997). Taken together, these domains comprise a body of feminist thought regarding patriarchy and the origin of women's oppression. The term 'patriarchy' comes from 'patriarch', an ancient word referring to Abraham, Isaac and Jacob, the founders of the Tribe of Israel, as told in the Book of Genesis. The contemporary meaning, however, does not 'refer to any individual men or even a collection of men' but to a society, or system of social organisation in which the values and interests of men are dominant (Volbrecht 2002, p. 167). Feminist politics traverses several intellectual traditions, including liberal, socialist, Marxist, radical, multiculturalist, cultural, global, psychoanalytical, existential, ecofeminist and postmodern. Discussing each of these in any detail would take us beyond the bounds of this chapter, but they can be examined in groups. For liberal feminists, oppression of women follows from not having access to the same opportunities as men. This can be remedied by instituting procedures that ensure equal opportunity for women. Equal access to the same educational, employment and career trajectories as men would eliminate discrimination based on gender. Radical feminists see the root cause of women's subordination in patriarchy, that is, in sociological terms and as a system of organisation that controls sexuality and reproduction. Gender-based economic arrangements are the origins for Marxists and socialist feminists, and child rearing practices for

psychoanalytical feminists. (Rosemarie Tong (1996) has written of the different kinds of questions and concerns that would be raised in a specific health care ethics context by liberal, radical and cultural feminists.)

Epistemology is the theory of knowledge. It is an area of philosophy concerned with the questions: who can be a 'knower'; what kinds of things can be known; and what are the standards that justify beliefs being legitimated as knowledge (Harding 1987, p. 3)? Feminist epistemology provides an account of knowledge differing from the standard view in western thought that posits that pure, objective knowledge is possible (Schott 1993). Taking the name of the ancient Greek philosopher and mathematician, Archimedes, the traditional view holds that there is a point (what has come to be known as an Archimedean point) that stands outside of what is known and can render a pure, objective knowledge. Rather like the photographs of the earth taken from space, the knower is conceived to have a privileged place from which knowledge is obtained and held to be true. Throughout the history of western thought, there have been two such places: religion and science or reason. With the former, God is the ultimate source of true knowledge. Developments in science and various historical factors began to challenge this view, so that Galileo marked a major shift in western thought. In proposing a new account of the physical universe, he challenged the Church's notion as the final arbiter of knowledge. Reason, and subsequently science rather than faith and Church authority, became the arbiters of knowledge.

In the history of thought, several alternative views of knowledge have followed in response, including, among others, phenomenology, critical theory and feminist thought. These alternative views share the perspective that knowledge can never be pure or never entirely objective, and that each knower is situated in a given place, time and set of circumstances. Feminist epistemologists are particularly concerned with women as knowers and, thus, with the experiences of women (Code 1991). Yet, even the category of 'women' is problematic for feminists because women inhabit a variety of different worlds with differing social conditions, languages, etc. Women in affluent, industrialised societies of European origin will have had quite different experiences from those of Pacific Islanders and indigenous peoples of North America or sub-Saharan Africa. For feminist theorists, it is not that knowledge is not possible, but that it is positional or situated knowledge.

Ontology is that branch of philosophy concerned with the nature or essence of things or existence. Ontology seeks to answer such questions as: what is time, space, a dog, a human being, a woman? In terms of ethics, ontology is relevant because it defines the entity of concern that influences how one should and does act towards and respond to others. Most feminist theorists see the nature of the human being as one whose identity is formed in relation to others, including family, friends, communities of place (where one lives) or communities of choice (those whom one chooses, for example, the gay community or a labour organisation), nations, and so forth. Because these relationships are significant for self-identity, formation of values, and ways of thinking about the self, the other, and the world, human beings are not autonomous in the way that political theory usually presents them. In contrast to the frequently claimed meaning of autonomy as atomistic and individualisitic, feminists refer to relational autonomy (Mackenzie and Stoljar 2000, Sherwin 1998), the self–other relation (Whitbeck 1984), the social self (Barclay 2000), and the autokoenonous self, or the self in community (Hoagland 1988).

Politics, epistemology and ontology are relevant to ethics of any approach but they are especially so to a feminist approach because feminist understandings challenge the traditional categories and lead to alternative views of moral reasoning and ethics.

MORAL REASONING AND ETHICAL DOMAINS

Morality is a practical matter concerning how to live in a complex and uncertain world. Moral reasoning is concerned with how we think about the practical moral problems encountered in the world. Persons, regardless of gender, reason in response to moral challenges. Yet, models of moral reasoning have come largely from male philosophers and psychologists, including Aristotle, Thomas Aquinas, and Immanuel Kant. Kant (1785) wrote during the early period of the Enlightenment and although he retained many Christian ideas, he made a major shift in grounding his moral philosophy in reason rather than faith (Taylor 1985). This secularised morality in that making moral judgements and living a moral life were open to any person of reason and did not require God as a foundation.

Kant's moral philosophy was occasioned largely in response to David Hume, for whom morality was a matter of sympathy, by which he meant one's capacity to be affected by the suffering of others. Kant's approach effectively eliminated emotions from moral motivation and reasoning. The formulations of the categorical imperative, the core of Kant's moral theory, are characterised by universality, impartiality and abstraction. Kantian moral philosophy and psychology came together in Lawrence Kohlberg's work (1958). Kohlberg (1976), who was a student of Jean Piaget, described the now famous stages of moral development from his 20-year longitudinal study of 84 boys. In this model of moral reasoning, abstract rules and principles, fairness and reciprocity, and duties and obligations for self and society are emphasised.

Kohlberg's student, Carol Gilligan (1982), challenged the male bias in his work by studying women and found 'a different voice' in women's descriptions of themselves and their moral lives. Gilligan referred to this different voice as an 'ethic of care' as opposed to Kohlberg's 'ethic of justice'. She discovered that the moral orientation of care was focused on the care and nurturing of self and others, the alleviation of hurt and suffering, the maintenance of relationships, and the contextual details of concrete situations involving particular individuals. Gilligan's 'ethic of care' was followed by that of Nel Noddings (1984). Like Gilligan, Noddings compared a caring approach with a justice or principle-based approach. She argued that a principle-based approach usually describes the relation between an individual person and certain principles that guide him or her toward an ideal life. In contrast, she argued, that relational ethics, like an ethic of care, concentrated more upon the moral quality of relationships than upon individuals. The 'ethic of care' and the 'ethic of justice' are now familiar concepts in both general and health care ethics. Feminist philosophers and nursing theorists have responded in different ways but, in order to appreciate the different strands this has taken, it is necessary to look at the domains of ethical experience.

The ethical world consists of three domains: injunctions, virtues and ways or forms of life, also referred to as cultural ethos (Pojman 1990, Yearley 1990). Yearley provides a brief but excellent description of these domains. Injunctions are 'those moral prohibitions or commands that people in a culture think present inviolable rights, duties, or claims' (p 8). 'They protect the bare necessities needed if human life is to function adequately' (p. 9). Typically, they are viewed as being universal or applicable to all societies. In traditional societies, injunctions are generally seen as reflecting a religious world-view, while in western societies since Kant, they are seen as the products of rational reflection or reasoning. Bernard Williams (1985) calls this domain the 'morality system' and it is this domain that has, for the most part, occupied moral philosophers since Kant. These approaches continue to look at rational justification and determination of injunctions, what feminist philosopher Margaret Urban Walker (1998, 2002) refers to as the theoretical-juridical model of morality and moral theory.

Virtues are 'ideals of human excellence' (Yearley 1990, p. 3), 'accounts of the character and interactions of practical reason, the emotions, and dispositions' (p. 5), 'a disposition to act, desire, and feel that involves the exercise of judgment and leads to a recognizable human excellence or instance of human flourishing' (p.

13). In any given society, virtues are hierarchically ordered. A contemporary feminist definition holds that virtues are 'linked capacities to attend, describe, inquire relevantly, feel appropriately, and respond reliably to situations of a certain kind' (Walker 1992, p. 32). In the ancient world, virtues were central to the ethical life but they fell by the wayside after the Medieval period. A renewed interest in them has developed over the past 40 years, since publication of an article by the British philosopher, G E M (Elizabeth) Anscombe (1958), who argued that ethics needed to attend to our moral psychologies and the role of emotions and feelings in our ethical lives. Emotions are central to feminist philosophers.

Ways or forms of life, 'the ethos of a culture', as Yearley (1990, p. 9) explains it, are both the vaguest and the most complex of the areas. This domain consists of deliberately chosen, explicit ideals as well as ideals of which we are essentially unaware and that are not deliberately chosen. A way of life is essentially how life is organised. These ideals are manifest in the ways in which we organise and structure society to inform society's cultural beliefs, attitudes and actions. Some would argue that ethical conflicts are the result of how we organise society (Chambliss 1996, Orgel 1983). A way of life structures gender and sex roles, class and race relationships, the division of labour within a society, the distribution of status, and what knowledge and skills are privileged; it is thus related to how power is exercised within a given society.

These domains are linked in that 'forms of life are protected by injunctions and picked out by the virtues' (Yearley 1990, p. 8). An especially close link exists between the virtues and a way of life. Virtues depend on a particular way of life in which they are embedded (Yearley 1990). One particular ethos will prize certain virtues over others. Ways of life differ not only between societies but also change over time. For example, in ancient Greece, manhood characterised by physical prowess was suited to a warrior culture. Yearley gives the example that virtues needed for a revolutionary political commitment are not compatible with a life characterised by decent usefulness and normal family loyalty. Typically, social scientists and historians have examined a way of life, leaving the injunctions to the moral philosophers, until the feminists came, that is. Feminist theorists have shown just how connected these domains are, particularly virtue and a way of life.

FEMINIST ETHICS

At the outset it is important to emphasise that 'feminist' does not mean hating men or being sexist. Being feminist is about a commitment to creating a world in which all people are free to flourish. Given the centrality of feminist concerns with the moral wrongs of oppression and domination, it is noteworthy that feminist ethics addresses these wrongs in all of their manifestations, including those of race, class, disability, sexual orientation and so forth.

In our view, the ethic of care is most closely related to the ethical domain of virtue or character. We believe this because of the emphasis it places on those aspects of the person that foster moral emotions and motivation, and serve to maintain the well-being of vulnerable others in our everyday lives.

Annette Baier (1985a, 1986) argues that what women want in a moral theory is exactly what Gilligan has begun: attention to the sustaining of relationships necessary to human life. She develops this further by suggesting that the most fruitful key concept may not be care, but rather trust. Yet this trust is not limited to the trust of the makers of a social contract. In her masterful contrast of the moralities of Hume and Kant, Baier (1987) highlights the importance of a morality based in human affection (Hume 1777) and the implications of such an understanding for a morality between non-autonomous, non-equal parties. She wonders if perhaps feminists have overlooked the relevance of Hume for understanding morality from a feminist perspective. Although Robin Schott (1993) does not compare Hume and Kant, her analysis of why Kant has been so successful in western civilization would suggest that Hume is far too

concerned with emotions, traditionally thought to be a downfall of women.

This concern with and attention to emotions is a critical feature of much of feminist theory in general (Boddington 1988, Code 1988, Held 1993, Jaggar 1989, Nussbaum 1995, 2001, Olesen 1990). Alison Jaggar points out that our values are rooted in our emotional lives and argues for the importance of this for our knowledge as well as our morality. It seems that a recognition of the role of emotions in our lives puts people back at the centre of philosophical inquiry. This centrality of particular people and their context is pivotal to feminist theory, even if there is acknowledgement that such a position cannot account for all human relationships (Purdy 1989, Stocker 1987, Tronto 1989). According to Walker (1989), 'current philosophical practice still largely views ethics as the search for moral knowledge, and moral knowledge as comprising universal moral formulae and the theoretical justification of these' (p. 15). Yet Seyla Benhabib (1987) offers a cogent demonstration of how the universal and abstract 'other' in the Kantian and Rawlsian positions is not a person at all, thereby rendering such positions incoherent. Thus Walker (1989) calls for 'an alternative moral epistemology, a very different way of identifying and appreciating the forms of intelligence which define responsible moral consideration' (p. 16). The central features of such an alternative epistemology include the understanding of particular persons in particular contexts, where context is taken to be a given relationship with a specific history, identity and emotional definition, and which are united by narratives. Also essential to Walker's alternative epistemology is 'the ability to communicate among persons involved or affected' (p. 18).

Although feminists agree that moral life requires a focal concern with interdependence, emotions and particularity, many are highly critical of these elements associated with an ethic of care in the absence of attention to the political, which is part of a form of life. These critics have indicated that, while an ethic of care may describe well the moral orientation of many women, it fails to examine critically the origins of this orientation and also its impact on the welfare of society, particularly women. The ethic of care may grow out of and may perpetuate women's unrecognised and often exploited caregiving, leading to further powerlessness and oppression. Its focus on intimate others could also lead to dangerous forms of partiality that ignore the needs of unknown others (Card 1988, 1990, Hoagland 1990, Houston 1992, Mullett 1988, Peter and Morgan 2001, Shogan 1992, Tong 1996, Tronto 1993). In addition, caring and caring practices, like caring for the sick and dying and the education of children, are also devalued by the dominant culture, making an ethic of care vulnerable to the same devaluation. Consequently, some writers have referred to an ethic of care as a 'feminine ethic' in contrast to a 'feminist ethic' (Sherwin 1992, Liaschenko 1993a, Jaggar 1995). In their view, a political perspective is required in order for an ethic to be considered feminist. Tong (1997) emphasises this by contrasting these perspectives as an 'ethic of care' and an 'ethic of power' respectively.

BOTH CARE AND POWER

In our view, philosopher Peta Bowden (1997, 2000) has made the most forceful (persuasive) argument that a feminine and a feminist ethics can be reconciled. In her in-depth study of caring, Bowden (1997) argued that ethics 'is a continuous process of mutual responses and adjustments' (p. 4) within particular contexts of actual people and real time, a theme that runs through feminist ethics (Baier 1985b, Liaschenko 1993b, Sherwin 1992, Walker 1998, 2002, Warren 1989). The very complexity and contextual nature of 'an actual morality' (Baier 1985b, p. 224) makes plain that no single moral concept, theory or judgement can resolve a given ethical issue once and for all (Bowden 1997, Held 1984, Liaschenko 2001). This is also true for an ethic of care. Bowden's strategy for understanding caring was a detailed exploration in a variety of contexts: mothering, nursing, friendship and citizenship. We discuss nursing specifically. Although Bowden drew on the work of several theorists for her study of caring in nursing, we

discuss only: Patricia Benner (1984) (including Benner and Wrubel (1989)) and Anne Bishop and John Scudder (1990). Bowden considers these authors to be exemplary in their argument for care, but concludes that they ultimately fail because they are limited in their ability to address feminist concerns.

Although the book, *From Novice to Expert* (Benner 1984), is not explicitly identified as ethics, it gives rich descriptions of nursing practice, demonstrating the contextual nature of actual clinical practice. It also richly describes the 'perceptual awareness', 'discretionary judgment', embodied intelligence, and emotional attentiveness to the person in excellent nursing (Bowden 1997). In *The Primacy of Caring*, Patricia Benner and Judith Wrubel (1989) elaborate on the healing relationships in nursing practice by exploring the meanings of personhood and the meanings of the illness to the person. According to Bowden (1997), even though Benner is aware of the constraints on nursing practice, nonetheless she 'slides over the complexity and immensity of the disempowering structural relations in which clinical nursing is enmeshed' (p. 120). Bowden (1997) argues that Benner's 'concern for structural impacts on caring is deflected with morale-raising talk of the special values of nursing care' (p. 121). The result is that:

Without a counterbalancing perspective that takes the realities of its deformations seriously, however, her account runs the risk of affirming structural relations which in contemporary North America, at least, often endorse and encourage the exploitation of nurses' capacities and hold them personally responsible for the failures of nursing care. (Bowden 1997, p. 122)

Bishop and Scudder (1990) begin with the recognition that nurses occupy an 'in-between' position in the institutional network of patients, physicians and management. The fact that health care requires a high level of collaboration between multiple parties renders nurses in the 'in-between' position ideally situated to enact ethically significant caring. This caring 'is characterized by the ethical potential to communicate between different members of the 'team' and to encourage co-operation and accommodation among those involved' (Bowden 1997, p. 126). Bowden (1997) sees their emphasis on the communal practice as a counter to the emphasis on rights and autonomy in health care but argues that 'they assume a level of communal solidarity and 'in-between' privilege that seems to overlook the widespread conflict and dissatisfaction that is such an outstanding feature of nursing practice in contemporary western institutions' (p. 127).

As Bowden (1997) sees it, nurses are 'roundly chastised for their failure to understand the inherent co-operative nature of their caring and its value' (p. 127). She concludes her analysis of Bishop and Scudder by saying:

In the light of disabling ideological and material forces, the claim that the ethical possibilities of nursing are centred in the obligation "to sustain excellent practice in the face of unreasonable demands which deny the legitimate authority of nurses", is highly problematic. (Bowden 1997, p. 128)

We have quoted extensively from Bowden (1997) in order to show readers the extent to which she views the call to care by Benner, and by Bishop and Scudder, to be faulty and inadequate. Yet Bowden (2000) argues that such a feminine ethic of care can be reconciled with a feminist ethic that necessarily entails institutional critique. An ethos of an ethic of care is a cultural climate in which ethically successful relationships are instituted and maintained. These relationships are characterised by responsiveness, mutuality, reciprocity, trust and so forth. Critical to such an ethos is one in which there is caring for those who are less, as well as more, vulnerable. Bowden recognises that clinical settings are constituted by networks of formal and informal organisations, hierarchically structured, and mediated by professional organisations and regulatory bodies. She therefore acknowledges that 'the conventionally understood language of care has a decidedly odd ring' (Bowden 2000, p. 44). She sees the institutional relations of clinical settings as involving: (1) state, political, economic, and high-tech relations; (2) relations with the medical profession; (3) relations with the clinical bureaucracy; and (4) professional nursing relations. Nonetheless, she maintains, 'the ethics of care can be seen as underwriting the characteristics of a desirable ethical culture, potential in every relationship no matter where the weight of vulnerabilities lies' (p. 44).

FEMINIST ETHICS, NURSING ETHICS AND DOMAINS OF ETHICAL EXPERIENCE

Like Bowden, we believe that the enactment of caring relationships is an essential good for human life, but we are less convinced that an ethic of care can do the work that Bowden believes that it can. We want to approach our scepticism by looking at the domains of ethical experience and how they relate. In our view, it makes sense to think of 'care' and 'caring' people as falling within the domain of virtue. To be a 'caring' individual is to be a certain kind of person, to hold certain values, and to evaluate oneself and one's actions in relation to these values. The origins and meanings of values have complex relationships with the world and its inhabitants. Each of us is born into a culture and a way of life that is mediated by relationships along a continuum from intimate or local to impersonal or global (Liaschenko 1997).

Bowden recognises the implications of a cultural ethos, arguing for care as the central moral value because it would result in ethically successful relationships. We do not disagree. Whereas Bowden moves beyond the 'individual,' she has shown that major theorists do not, or do so in such a limited way as to render them ineffective. In our view, these theorists are essentially conservative. Although we see Bowden as attempting to move beyond this conservatism, we find the following problems. First, care restricts the domain of moral action to the interpersonal. To be fair, Bowden attempts to unite an ethic of care and an ethic of power in a clinical setting that one would expect to be primarily about interpersonal relationships. However, even here, this is not always the case. An ethic of care is a set of practices, values and thinking that responds to others in personal relationships. This makes sense in that there is a proximity that allows certain actions to take place so that the care can actually be enacted. Yet, there are situations in which this cannot take place. There are domains or arenas of action in which the moral agent, in this case the nurse, cannot act in such a way that care can be enacted.

For example, a nurse who is working in a substance abuse treatment centre for injection drug users can be assumed to be knowledgeable, not only about the medical aspects of addiction but also about the everyday world and lives of injection drug users. From extensive experience involving careful listening, she knows the social circumstances and patterns of drug use. She believes that needle exchanges would work to decrease the risk of AIDS and hepatitis C because the people she works with have told her they would use such a programme. Yet, she is not at liberty to issue clean syringes for her clients; this is outside of her domain of possible action because that is a political action that occurs at a different level of social interaction. If she were to do this, she would violate norms of the profession and the community at large. To enact this practice, she must work politically to make this happen. Much of this work may involve interpersonal relationships in attempting to educate people, but a significant aspect of this work may be the casting of a vote for a political candidate who supports needle exchanges, or voting for the practice directly in a referendum. The outcome of this political action will either reinforce existing norms or create new ones.

Contemporary social life in the West, and specifically in North America, is essentially organised via institutions, via highly bureaucratised, increasingly privatised and corporatised political economies under advanced capitalism. 'Institution' in this sense, is more than a building or even a network of action such as a health care system involving several hospitals, outpatient clinics, home care divisions, and so forth. By institutions we mean linked networks of such organising features as professional structures, governmental and other regulatory bodies, and accrediting bodies. An advertisement placed some years ago by the American Medical Association in several magazines typically found in physician waiting rooms pictured a line of ducks with the words 'quack, quack, quack' written below it. The advertisement said something about seeking care from a nurse practitioner; the connection was unmistakable. The reason for the advertisement was actually quite understandable; it represented a threat owing to an actual or perceived turf war.

We can appreciate the self-interests of groups, others as well as our own. Nevertheless, we make no excuses for the blatant hostility expressed towards nurse practitioners in that advertisement. Our point is that no amount of interpersonal caring could have been successful in having it withdrawn; that took organised action from a representative organisation such as the American Nurses Association. Similarly, when nurses were being laid off in large numbers in Alberta, Canada, physicians were silent about the implication for nurses, patients and health care in general, until they started losing *their* jobs. We wish to be very clear here; we are not pointing to individuals, but to organisations representing groups, in this case, physicians. Interpersonal relationships may go a long way towards reaching mutual understanding and respect, but they are not sufficient in situations such as these.

The TV show, 'The Nightingales' was a 'sitcom' that portrayed nurses as sex objects. Both the TV show and the advertisement were withdrawn after forceful lobbying and attention on the part of the American Nurses Association. Although it may be the case that individual nurses enacted caring relationships with physicians and others, it can hardly be claimed that it was sufficient for changing such blatantly sexist and hostile messages. There is a plausible argument that, if those responsible for conceiving, initiating and seeing through these projects had had caring relationships with nurses, the programme might never have reached the public domain. The domain of action of any individual nurse, even every nurse acting in concert, requires a range of relationships beyond the interpersonal, where mutuality and reciprocity are central.

Bowden (2000) is right to be concerned about the use of reductive language, such as normalcy, sickness, autonomy and dependency. These words quickly become useless for anything other than unreasoned acceptance of routinised action that keeps everyone under the illusion that everything we do in our health care institutions makes sense. The most sceptical part of us agrees that it may indeed make a great deal of sense, but often not to nurses at the bedside. Where we differ from Bowden is that we see the language of care as equally reductive. 'Dare to Care' says the most recent advertisement on local American TV, in an attempt to recruit people into nursing. Such advertisements do nothing to reveal the complexity of nursing work, or to acknowledge that some people who seek to become nurses may simply need or desire the advantages that nursing provides, like a means to pay the mortgage. We know that this will be received as 'blasphemous', but it does point to the way that caring has become an ideology, even a technology, as Margarete Sandelowski (2000) claims.

Finally, we agree with Bowden (2000) that 'professional educational practices that isolate ethical insight from institutional power effects by embracing either the feminine version of care ethics or the bioethics model' (p. 38) are inadequate. We would say again only that these are forces that lie outside individual nurses and beyond the profession. If nurses have taken up these educational practices to a larger extent than others have, it is plausible to ask what it was about the earlier cultural ethos of nursing that led to this. What did gender have to do with it? What did class have to do with it? For what virtues did such an ethos select? A feminine ethic of care, perhaps?

To say that certain cultural practices lie beyond the domain of action of individual nurses is not meant to convey some moral nihilism—that nothing can be done—on our part. A growing body of nursing ethics scholarship has paid close attention to identifying and transforming powerful institutional structures. Since Anne Davis and Mila Aroskar's (1978) publication that identified organisational and social constraints inherent in the employee status of nurses, there has been wide recognition of the politically situated nature of nurses' moral agency. Ronald Yarling and Beverly McElmurry (1986) take a very strong position, arguing that nurses are not free to be moral because of their conflicting obligations to patients, employers, physicians, nursing administrators, and their own moral convictions. They recommend a social ethic that would seek to reform the structures and policies of institutions, much like a feminist ethic that expressly focuses on the need not only to identify oppression but also to transform society. Patricia Rodney and Rosalie Starzomski (1993) also describe how nurses' structural and interpersonal work environment can lead to moral distress in nurses because their capacity to fulfil their responsibilities is jeopardised. In a more recent publication, Colleen Varcoe and Patricia Rodney (2002) not only identify the structural constraints nurses face through administrative policies, procedures and practices, but also add to the notion of constraint by showing how they can also exist ideologically, such as through an ideology of scarcity that leads nurses to believe that quality care is no longer affordable owing to current fiscal realities (Ceci and McIntyre 2001).

In our own work (Liaschenko 1993a, Peter 1998, 2000, Peter and Morgan 2001), we have argued that, while care is necessary for nursing ethics, it is not sufficient. Nursing ethics concerns need to be politically situated and nursing ethics could benefit from alternative ethical concepts, such as trust. Furthermore, injunctions in the form of principles are also needed to ensure that nursing relationships are not overly idealised and that the potential for evil is recognised. The challenge remains, however, to draw these various domains together to form a comprehensive, yet coherent, moral approach. A feminist approach has much to contribute to this endeavour.

REFERENCES

Anscombe G E M 1958 Modern moral philosophy. Philosophy 33 (124): 1–19

Baier A 1985a What do women want in a moral theory? Nouse 19 (1): 53–65

Baier A 1985b Postures of the mind. University of Minnesota Press, Minneapolis, MN, p. 207-227

Baier A 1986 Trust and antitrust. Ethics 96 (2): 231–260

Baier A 1987 Hume, the women's moral theorist? In: Kittay E F, Meyers D T (eds) Women and moral theory. Rowman and Littlefield, Totowa, NJ, p. 37–55

Barclay L 2000 Autonomy and the social self. In: Mackenzie C, Stoljar N (eds) Relational autonomy: feminist perspectives on autonomy, agency, and the social self. Oxford University Press, New York, p. 52–71

Bell L A 1993 Rethinking ethics in the midst of violence. Rowman and Littlefield, Lanham, MD

Benhabib S 1987 The generalized and the concrete other: the Kohlberg-Gilligan controversy and moral theory. In: Kittay E F, Meyers D T (eds) Women and moral theory. Rowman and Littlefield, Totowa, NJ, p. 155–177

Benner P 1984 From novice to expert. Addison-Wesley, Menlo Park, CA

Benner P, Wrubel J 1989 The primacy of caring: stress and coping in health and illness. Addison-Wesley, Menlo Park, CA

Bishop A H, Scudder J R 1990 The practical, moral and personal sense of nursing: a phenomenological philosophy of practice. State University of New York Press, Albany, NY

Boddington P R 1988 The issue of women's philosophy. In: Griffiths M, Whifford M (eds) Feminist perspectives in philosophy. Indiana University Press, Indianapolis, IN, p. 205-223

Bowden P 1997 Caring: gender-sensitive ethics. Routledge, London

Bowden P 2000 An 'ethic' of care in clinical settings: encompassing 'feminine' and 'feminist' perspectives. Nursing Philosophy 1 (1): 36–49

Brennan S 1999 Recent work in feminist ethics. Ethics 109 (4): 858–893

Browning Cole E, Coultrap-McQuin S 1992 Explorations in feminist ethics: theory and practice. Indiana University Press, Bloomington, IN

Card C 1988 Women's voices and ethical ideals: must we mean what we say? Ethics 99 (1): 125–135

Card C 1990 Caring and evil. Hypatia 5 (1): 101–108

Card C 1991 Feminist ethics. University of Kansas Press, Lawrence, KS

Ceci C, McIntyre M 2001 A quiet crisis in nursing: developing our capacity to hear. Nursing Philosophy 2 (2): 1–9

Chambliss D F 1996 Beyond caring: hospitals, nurses and the social organization of ethics. University of Chicago Press, Chicago, IL

Code L 1988 Experience, knowledge and responsibility. In: Griffiths M, Whifford M (eds) Feminist perspectives in philosophy. Indiana University Press, Indianapolis, IN, p. 187–204

Code L 1991 What can she know? Feminist theory and the construction of knowledge. Cornell University Press, Ithaca, NY

Davis A, Aroskar M 1978 Ethical dilemmas and nursing practice. Appleton-Century-Crofts, Norwalk, CT

Diamant A 1997 The red tent. St Martin's Press, New York

Gilligan C 1982 In a different voice: psychological theory and women's development. Harvard University Press, Cambridge, MA

Harding S (ed) 1987 Feminism and methodology. Indiana University Press, Bloomington, IN

Held V 1984 Rights and goods – justifying social action. Free Press, New York

Held V 1993 Feminist morality: transforming culture, society and politics. University of Chicago Press, Chicago, IL

Hoagland S 1988 Lesbian ethics. Institute of Lesbian Studies, Palo Alto, CA

Hoagland S 1990 Some concerns about Nel Noddings' caring. Hypatia 5 (1): 109–114

Houston B 1992 Prolegomena to future caring. In: Shogan D (ed) A reader in feminist ethics. Canadian Scholars' Press, Toronto, p. 109–128

Hume D 1777 Enquiries concerning human understanding and concerning the principles of morals, 3rd edn (Selby-Bigge L A (ed) 1989) Clarendon Press, Oxford

Jaggar A 1989 Love and knowledge: emotion in feminist epistemology. In: Jaggar A, Bordo S (eds) Gender, body, knowledge: feminist reconstructions of being and knowing. Rutgers University Press, New Brunswick, NJ, p. 145–171

Jaggar A 1995 Toward a feminist conception of moral reasoning. In: Sterba J, Machan T, Jaggar A et al (eds) Morality and social justice. Rowman and Littlefield, Lanham, MD, p. 115–146

Kant I 1785 Foundations of the metaphysics of morals and what is enlightenment. (White Beck L trans 1959). Macmillan, New York

Kohlberg L 1958 The development of modes of thinking and choices in years 10 to 16 [dissertation]. University of Chicago, Chicago, IL

Kohlberg L 1976 Moral stages and moralization: the cognitive-developmental approach. In: Lickona T (ed) Moral development and behavior: theory, research and social issues. Holt, Rinehart and Winston, New York, p. 31–53

Lengerman P, Niebrugge-Brantley J 1988 Contemporary feminist theory. In: Ritzer G (ed) Sociological theory, 2dn edn. Alfred A Knopf, New York, p. 400–443

Liaschenko J 1993a Feminist ethics and cultural ethos: revisiting a nursing debate. Advances in Nursing Science 15 (4): 71–81

Liaschenko J 1993b Faithful to the good: morality and philosophy in nursing practice [dissertation]. University of California, San Francisco, CA

Liaschenko J 1997 Ethics and the geography of the nurse-patient relationship: spatial vulnerabilities and gendered space. Scholarly Inquiry for Nursing Practice 11 (1): 45–59

Liaschenko J 2001 Nursing work, housekeeping issues, and the moral geography of home care. In: Weisstub D N, Thomasma D C, Gauthier S, Tomossy G F (eds) Aging: caring for our elders. Kluwer Academic Press, Dordrecht, p. 123–137

Mackenzie C, Stoljar N 2000 (eds) Relational autonomy: feminist perspectives on autonomy, agency, and the social self. Oxford University Press, New York

Mullett S 1988 Shifting perspectives: a new approach to ethics. In: Code L, Mullett S, Overall C (eds) Feminist perspectives: philosophical essays on method and morals. University of Toronto, Toronto, p. 109–126

Noddings N 1984 Caring: a feminine approach to ethics and education. University of California Press, Berkley, CA

Nussbaum M C 1995 Emotions and women's capabilities. In: Nussbaum M C, Glover J (eds) Women, culture and development: a study of human capabilities. Clarendon Press, Oxford, p. 360–395

Nussbaum M C 2001 Upheavals of thought: the intelligence of emotions. Cambridge University Press, New York

Olesen V 1990 The neglected emotions: a challenge to medical sociology [plenary address] Procedures of the 20th Annual British Sociological Association Conference, Edinburgh

Orgel G S 1983 They have no right to know: the nurse and the terminally ill patient. In: Murphy C P, Hunter H (eds) Ethical problems in the nurse-patient relationship. Allyn and Bacon, Boston, MA, p. 123–136

Peter E 1998 Trust: a feminist ethic for nursing practice [dissertation]. University of Toronto, Toronto

Peter E 2000 The politicization of ethical knowledge: feminist ethics as a basis for home care nursing research. Canadian Journal of Nursing Research 32 (2): 103–118

Peter E, Morgan K 2001 Explorations of a trust approach for nursing ethics. Nursing Inquiry 8 (1): 3–10

Pojman L 1990 Ethics: discovering right and wrong. Wadsworth, Belmont, CA

Purdy L M 1989 Feminists healing ethics. Hypatia 4 (2): 9–14

Rodney P, Starzomski R 1993 Constraints on the moral agency of nurses. Canadian Nurse 89 (9): 23–26

Sandelowski M 2000 Devices and desires: gender, technology, and American nursing. University of North Carolina Press, Chapel Hill, NC

Sherwin S 1998 A relational approach to autonomy in health care. In: Sherwin S (ed) The politics of women's health; exploring agency and autonomy. Temple University Press, Philadelphia, PA, p. 19–47

Schott R 1993 From cognition to eros: a critique of the Kantian paradigm. Pennsylvania State University Press, University Park, PA

Shogan D 1992 Feminist ethics for strangers. In: Shogan D (ed) A reader in feminist ethics. Canadian Scholars' Press, Toronto, p. 171–184

Stocker M 1987 Duty and friendship: towards a synthesis of Gilligan's contrastive moral concepts. In: Kittay E F, Meyers D T (eds) Women and moral theory. Rowman and Littlefield, Totowa, NJ, p. 56–68

Taylor R 1985 Ethics, faith and reason. Prentice-Hall, Englewood Cliffs, NJ

Tong R 1996 An introduction to feminist approaches to bioethics: unity in diversity. Journal of Clinical Ethics 7 (1): 13–29

Tong R 1997 Feminist approaches to bioethics. Westview Press, Boulder, CO

Tronto J C 1989 Women and caring: what can feminists learn about morality from caring? In: Jaggar A, Bordo S (eds) Gender, body, knowledge: feminist reconstructions of being and knowing. Rutgers University Press, New Brunswick, NJ, p. 172–187

Tronto J C 1993 Moral boundaries: a political argument for an ethic of care. Routledge, New York

Varcoe C, Rodney P 2002 Constrained agency: the social structure of nurses' work. In: Bolaria B S, Dickinson H D (eds) Health, illness and health care in Canada. Nelson Thomson Learning, Toronto, p. 102–128

Volbrecht R M 2002 Nursing ethics: communities in dialogue. Prentice Hall, Upper Saddle River, NJ

Walker M U 1989 Moral understandings: alternative 'epistemology' for a feminist ethics. Hypatia 4 (2): 15–28

Walker M U 1992 Feminism, ethics, and the question of theory. Hypatia 7 (3): 23–38

Walker M U 1998 Moral understandings: a feminist study in ethics. Routledge, New York

Walker M U 2002 Morality in practice: a response to Claudia Card and Lorraine Code. Hypatia 17 (1): 174–182

Warren V 1989 Feminist directions in medical ethics. Hypatia 42 (1): 73–87

Whitbeck C 1984 A different reality: feminist ontology. In: Gould C (ed) Beyond domination: new perspectives on women and philosophy. Rowman and Allanheld, Totowa, NJ, p. 24–88

Williams B 1985 Ethics and the limits of philosophy. Harvard University Press, Cambridge, MA

Yarling R R, McElmurry B J 1986 The moral foundation of nursing. Advances in Nursing Science 8 (2): 63–73

Yearley L H 1990 Mencius and Aquinas: theories of virtue and conceptions of courage. State University of New York Press, Albany, NY

Young I M 1990 Justice and the politics of difference. Princeton University Press, Princeton, NJ

5

Relational ethics: an action ethic as a foundation for health care*

Wendy Austin   Vangie Bergum   John Dossetor

Some of the reasons for this book's existence are articulated by the authors of this chapter, Wendy Austin, Vangie Bergum and John Dossetor, in their opening paragraphs. The general thrust of ethics teaching had become increasingly difficult to take on board, because teachers and students of any standing realised that the most important aspects of ethics—the relationships of the people involved—were too often neglected. This chapter makes a most valid contribution to the argument concerning why relationships are fundamental in all ethical understanding, dealings and decisions. Learning to hear what the people concerned are feeling, saying and thinking, and acting on this, is crucial if the outcome is to be such that people can not only live with it but be enhanced by what was done and decided.

WHAT IS RELATIONAL ETHICS?

Relational ethics is based on the assumption that ethical practice is situated in relationship. It is within the context of intricate, close-up relationships that health professionals determine how to be and how to act. The use of a relational approach as a foundation for health ethics means that, although the principles of ethics, practice standards, codes of conduct, procedural rules and policies are regarded as useful guides for ethical action, they are not considered an adequate basis for ethical practice. Acting

* The research upon which this chapter is based is described in full in: Bergum V, Dossetor J (in press) Relational ethics: the full meaning of respect. University Publishing, Hagerstown, MD

ethically is more than achieving the right resolution to moral dilemmas. It is more than good decision making when crises arise. Ethical practice is about commitment to the persons in one's care and the way in which one relates to them (Levine 1977).

A relational ethic stimulates a fundamental shift in our thinking about ethics. There is a move from concentration on solving the ethical 'problem' to asking the ethical question. The focus shifts from attention to the person as an individual (that is, a solitary bearer of rights) to recognition of the person as an interdependent agent (autonomous but situated in community with others, and thereby connected to others). Taking a relational ethics perspective means that one seeks to be sensitive to the particular care situation through the opening of dialogue between and among individuals, the consideration of intuitive responses to persons and issues, and an appreciation of the uncertainty inherent in human circumstances.

SITUATING RELATIONAL ETHICS IN THEORIES OF ETHICS

The metaphor of a coral reef has been used to show how different approaches to ethical knowledge build and develop on one another (Gadow 1999). Prior forms of knowledge provide a supporting structure for new life and growth. It is the moral theories of Kant, Rawls, Mills and others that have provided the underpinnings of contemporary ethical thinking for health care practice and can be understood as providing the structure for the relational approach to flourish. The principles used in ethical decision making (such as non-maleficience, beneficence, autonomy and justice) (Beauchamp and Childress 2001) build upon theories of personal rights and freedom, a concern for equality and fairness, and the importance of rationality. This philosophical structure alone has increasingly been found wanting as sufficient guidance for day-to-day ethical action, by practitioners and academics alike.

In the early 1980s Carol Gilligan (1982) led in the call for a new structure to ethics in which the essentiality of care, connection and respect was acknowledged. Recognition of human connection, it was argued, is as crucial to ethics as a right to autonomy. Although viewing patients as separate, rational and autonomous individuals is congruent with the scientific tradition of medicine and its expertise, this objective stance ignores the messy, ambiguous nature of everyday existence. It does not allow for attention to the fundamental relational dynamics of actual practice. The issues of power inherent in health care decisions and interventions, the vulnerability and dependency of those who are ill, and the role of emotion in authentic human experience, need to be taken up if our approach to decision making is to be ethical. Genuine intersubjectivity of health care relationships needs to be given attention.

Relational ethics is an attempt to create an ethic for health care that is grounded in our commitments to each other. Building upon both justice and care, the living branches of this ethic include a concept of personhood that values autonomy through connection, a recognition that sensitivity to ethical questions is as important as the ability to secure answers, and an awareness that our practice environments shape our moral responses. It is an action-orientated ethic, although sometimes the ethical action will be just 'being there'. Instead of doing as the familiar North American suggests, 'Don't just stand there, do something', a relational ethics approach asks one to consider the merits of the opposite: 'Don't just do something, stand there!' Relational ethics is about being with, as well as being for, the other.

THE RELATIONAL ETHICS PROJECT

The insights regarding relational ethics described in this chapter evolve from a research project situated at the John Dossetor Health Ethics Centre, University of Alberta, Canada. Funded by the Social Sciences and Humanities Research Council of Canada (1993–2001) and led by Vangie Bergum and John Dossetor, the Relational Ethics Project was an endeavour aimed at elucidating the ethical commitments required by everyday health care situations. It was recognised that the underpinnings of western bioethics—principles and rules that point to right action; virtues that point to right character; casuistry that points to prior cases and situational analysis; and caring that points to the need for attention to the particularity of persons and the compassion of care-givers' knowledge—must have further grounding. We need to consider such questions as: Can one be morally indifferent to relationships as long as principles are applied? Can one be morally indifferent to relationships as long as the virtues of people are defendable? (Veatch, 1998). If our answer is 'No', then we need to gain a better understanding of the nature of ethical connections in health care practice. In Phase One of the research, real clinical situations were considered. They were 'brought into the room', so to speak, by the use of videos, photographs and art, literature and personal testimony. For example, we heard the stories of Allison, a comatose woman whose family described their journey toward the decision to remove her feeding tube; of Dax, a young man with such severe burns that he begged to be allowed to die; and of K'aila, an infant whose parents, deciding against organ transplantation for his liver disease, had to struggle to keep him in their care. As the research discussions of such real-life stories were analysed, a description of relational ethics evolved. The results are currently being published (Bergum and Dossetor in press). In Phase Two of the project, three foci were selected to examine relational ethics further: genetic counselling, mental health care and health care teams. The results of this phase are forthcoming.

CORE ELEMENTS OF A RELATIONAL ETHIC

Revealed by this research were elements that seem essential to a relational ethic. These include: mutual respect, engagement, embodied knowledge, uncertainty or possibility, and attention to the environment. Mutual respect arises from the reality that we are fundamentally dependent on one another. Our experience, not only of the world but of ourselves, is shaped by the attitude of others towards us and by our attitude towards others (Løgstrup 1971). We are living in a global age, and the truth regarding our fundamental connection and interconnection is becoming strikingly apparent (Austin 2001). Moral actions are interpersonal actions. Ethical action, then, needs to start with an attempt to understand the other's situation, perspective and vulnerability. This understanding requires a true movement towards the other person and a movement toward genuine engagement. When this is not possible, the lack of real involvement needs to be recognised as the ethical issue it is. The element of embodiment calls for a healing of the split between mind and body, and for an integrative consciousness, so that scientific knowledge and human compassion are given equal status and the importance of emotion and feeling in ethical action is appropriately accredited. We need to recognise that facts are not value-free. Our ethical reflections and deliberations should not be carried out as if, through the use of rational thought, the world can be made simple (i.e. just black and white). The uncertainty inherent in human existence is thus acknowledged and should even be embraced. It is uncertainty that opens possibility to us. Relational ethics brings attention to the environment, to the moral space in which health care occurs. As practitioners we ask ourselves whether or not our environment allows us to practice in the way that we believe we should. Do our practice environments support the raising of ethical questions, even the difficult and thorny ones, about the kind of relationships we hold? What kind of an environment is needed in order to practice ethically and how do we achieve or acquire what we need? What if there is simply not enough time to establish a relationship? How long, in fact, does it take to establish a relationship?

Descriptions of three of the core elements (embodied knowledge, relational engagement, and mutual respect) illustrate aspects of a relational ethics approach to health care practice.

Embodied knowledge

Allison Brown, a vibrant, young married woman, became comatose as the result of a car accident on the way home from work one rainy night. Following months of intensive care without any signs of improvement, Allison's family brought her to an extended care facility near them. For the next four years, the family and trained volunteers provided care and stimulation to Allison. At the end of this time, they decided to remove Allison's feeding tube. When they did so, Allison died.

The moral decision to remove the feeding tube that kept Allison alive was not a discrete one, nor an easy one. It began when the family first decided to remain an active part of her life, to continue to be with her and support her. As they cared for her, other ethical decisions emerged, for instance, the decision to treat her as an equal, different now, but still a family member: a daughter, a sister, and a wife. The ethic that guided them, they said, did not evolve out of abstract principles, or from an idea of Allison's moral identity. It evolved as they faced everyday practicalities. The time came when they felt that Allison did not want to be in her body any more. 'We felt this intuitively', they told the research team. 'There was nothing behind her eyes.' This meant that an enormous decision was before them.

Each family member struggled over what to do, trying to understand their own conscience and reconcile it with Allison's expressed wishes. (Prior to her accident, Allison had read about Karen Ann Quinlan and asked her sister to 'pull her tube' if she was ever in similar circumstances.) There was a diversity of belief systems among the family—'we're talking Christians, Buddhists, New Agers, and an atheist thrown into the mix'—but their beliefs converged around the meaning of Allison's life and the act of her death. 'Our convergence was actually gentle and after talking and talking and talking about it, we finally all agreed. We felt that our decision was correct based on who we were and what we knew of Allison.' Allison's family found that removing her feeding tube was 'a spiritual act'. 'We felt that it was the most difficult decision that we would ever have to make in our lives and we asked for spiritual guidance, not only from ministers and priests, but most importantly from within ourselves.'

For Allison's family, the dignity of human persons (of being a person) seemed to dwell in the reality of relationship rather than in the property possessed by one of the parties, whether cognition, or moral agency (Smith 1992). Although there are ethicists who argue that cognitively-impaired people are not 'persons' (Kuhse 1999), this does not fit with the experience of many family members and health care professionals. The face of the patient before us is the face of a person. We are with them, present to them, and they to us, even when there is 'nothing behind [their] eyes'. A member of the research group noted that:

For health care professionals, human beings with severe brain injury or dementia are still someone's mother, or sister, or, at least, someone's child—they are not an 'it', an animal, or a 'hunk of something'.

The story of Allison, her family, and the professional staff and volunteers who cared for her, reveals crucial aspects of the relational space where we must dwell in health care. This is the space where we embrace both thinking and feeling, both objectivity and subjectivity, and both self and other. We are in this space together, despite difference and diversity, and it is here that we can discover an irreducible respect for each other as whole persons. Here, we can come to know one another. Here, we come to know ourselves.

The attention given to the quality of Allison's life and of her death heightened her family's experience of their relationship with her, within the family itself and with the health care professionals who were accompanying Allison to the end of her life. 'Our circle was then enlarged to include nurses, doctors, ethicists, ministers, priests, extended family, caregivers and volunteers. It was this small community that gave us support and encouragement. They knew what Allison's life was like for the last four years and they were there for her when she passed away.' There is no doubt that relational commitments can be tremendously burdensome, but it is within such commitments that we discover the heart of care-taking (Burt and Cowart 1998). It is here we find the foundation for ethical practice, as noted by one researcher:

We don't go in knowing and giving this perfect care. To be aware of that and then to move to a better level of care is being ethical. The reflection and the self-awareness are part of being ethical because the most ethical practice cannot happen by just being technically competent.

Embodiment is found in relational space. This space between body and mind, between self and other—referred to as a 'third space' (Bhabha, 1994) or a 'dialogical space' (Taylor 1993)—builds on the embodied reality of life as lived. In this relational space where dualities cease we draw upon all aspects of life: our rationality, our emotionality, our connection to each other, our differences between each other, and our grounding in the world. It is a space in which we address our own and others' pain and vulnerability; we are wholly in it. We are attached, not detached. We are engaged.

Relational engagement

Dax Cowart, a pilot home from Vietnam, received severe, body-covering burns in a tragic accident that killed his father. When he was found, he asked to die. He continued to ask to die in hospital. There, Dax's burn treatments occasioned pain so intense that he would scream until he passed out from exhaustion. This went on—the treatment and his pain—everyday for weeks. Dax lived.

Dax's story took place in the 1970s but it still speaks strongly to us today. During the Relational Ethics Research Project, a video was viewed in which Dax's burn treatment sessions had been recorded (Anonymous, 1985). In this video excerpt we recognise that Dax cannot see and is covered with disfiguring, painful burns. He screams loudly as the care-givers treat his terrible wounds. There is a radio blaring in the background (which actually dominates the whole space) as his care-givers talk to each other, not seeming to acknowledge Dax's pain. Dax cries for his care-givers to take care while they focus on their work. Throughout the video, and for years after these hospital events, Dax continues to argue for his right to stop his treatments. At that time, he begged to be allowed to die but his pleas brought no response.

Caring for a patient who is suffering is incredibly demanding. It challenges us in a fundamental way. When people say, 'I could never be a doctor; I could never be a nurse', it is this kind of demand to which they are referring. 'I couldn't take it', they mean. 'I can't bear to see terrible pain, vomit, blood, disfigurement...' How do practitioners 'bear it'? Distancing may be one way. We work to keep ourselves apart from the patients, separate from their anguish. We struggle not to allow their pain to touch us. We hold ourselves separate from suffering and from patients' misery. Being disengaged can be framed as being professional. We don't get 'too involved'; we learn to stay detached in an effort to be 'objective'. One of Dax's physician's says, 'I had trouble with the eye and hand.' Focusing on the body parts that he is trying to heal may allow this physician to use skilled techniques in precise and necessary ways. Could he pull away the dead, burned tissue so precisely if he allowed himself to listen to Dax's cries? Does professional expertise require the impersonal?

Although the ideology of modern medicine opposes connection (Schultz and Carnevale 1996), in order to remain objective and prevent emotional hurt for either professional or patient, a relational ethic recognises that both patient and professional lose thereby. A relational ethics argues that ethical professional practice requires the personal, the intersubjective. Practitioners need to be responsive and open to those in their care, and to cultivate a sensitivity that promotes genuine connection. Being professional means learning to be engaged, not disengaged, with those in our care. Perhaps a 'shared moment'—a

moment of being with him in his pain—would have helped to ease Dax's anguish. Engagement requires 'a personal responsiveness to the particular other' (Gadow 1999, p. 63). It requires that we try to see the person before us in a genuine way; it means being present *with* them, not merely present in the room.

Dax's pleas for death seemed to fall upon deaf ears. One time when he asked a nurse to help him to die, the nurse told him, 'I can't.' He was at that moment heard and given the answer: 'I can't.' The nurse responded to him from herself. His desire for an end to his suffering was there between them, real and known. Although she could not cause his death as he desired, she did not distance herself from his anguish. Her own vulnerability was revealed: 'I can't end it for you. I can't help in this way.' Expression of her vulnerability through engagement with Dax was not a negative trait to be avoided; rather, by acknowledging her vulnerability (that is, bringing her true humanity into the relationship) she acknowledged her emotions and the impact of power in her relationship with him. If health care professionals experience vulnerability, the power differential between professional and patient is lost, and the possibility of engagement is increased.

It is our ability and willingness to empathise with others, to see and share their world to the extent that we can, that awakens moral perception and gives it direction (Reynolds et al 2000, Vetlesen 1994). In this moral response we do not lose ourselves, but rather we can discover ourselves, and find our capabilities. It is not an easy thing to learn, but we need to explore ways to achieve it:

How could we stand very close to Dax in order to see him or to hear him or to understand what it is that's happening for him? By standing that close, we are vulnerable to immersion in his pain and his suffering. So the question is: How do we stay completely present and not fall back on all of our socially and culturally and psychologically acceptable coping methods? Methods that are at our disposal for self-protection, actions such as distancing, leaving, reducing him.

To act in an engaged way, both care-givers

and recipients of care need to be whole beings in what has been called person-directed attention (Dillon 1992). 'The obligation of caring for another human being involves becoming a certain kind of person – not merely doing certain things' (Carper 1978, p. 23). When Raymond Duff (1987) says that 'the secret of caring for the patient is caring for the patient' (p. 245), he is giving voice to that relational place, the ethical moment where people connect with each other through respect.

Mutual respect

K'aila was an infant with liver disease. His parents' refusal of a liver transplant for him stimulated an adversarial process that led to the parents escaping out-of-province with K'aila for fear that they would lose their son to Social Services authorities. K'aila's physician, who believed that the rejection of his expert advice unnecessarily denied his tiny patient the possibility of life, had asked that society, through its instrument, the Courts of Law, intervene. K'aila died in the arms of his parents at the age of 11 months. The Courts upheld the parents' decision.

The life and death of K'aila, as presented in the video, 'A Choice for K'aila' (Anonymous 1993), evokes the element of mutual respect in ethical health care practice by its apparent absence. The tragedy of this baby's disease was deepened by the actions that arose in response to it. Although everyone wanted what was best for this child, the means taken to assure this outcome increased pain and hardship for all concerned. The physician, who had 'successfully' treated other children like K'aila— they were alive years later—assumed that the only reasonable option was a transplant. He had the technology and the skill to save K'aila. How could he stand by and watch this baby die? K'aila's parents, on the other hand, had strong spiritual views about Nature and its rhythms and beliefs, shaped by an Aboriginal heritage. These beliefs were profoundly reflected in their everyday life. They felt that aggressive treatment with life-long medical supervision was not in their son's best interests, so they refused a transplant.

The physician was guided by the vision of his responsibilities to his little patient, filtered through the lens of the principles of autonomy, beneficence, non-maleficence and justice. This approach, based on cognitive rational analysis (Beauchamp and Childress 2001), could not encompass the emotional, situational or spiritual aspects of K'aila's circumstances. The parents came to their decision through what Paulette, K'aila's mother, called a 'whole person' model. Although an understanding of the relevant medical knowledge was important to their decision (they reviewed it until they felt they knew what a transplant would mean for their son), the heartfelt dimensions of love and feeling and a spiritual sense of the interconnection of life weighed significantly (Paulette 1993).

Although K'aila's best interests were the intent of both family and physician, respect for one another's points of view was a missing piece. The parents did not feel respected by the physician because they chose a palliative rather than an aggressive approach to their child's disease. The physician did not experience respect because the child was taken from his care to another province and another physician. Without mutual respect, the tragedy that surrounded K'aila's dying was deepened, not eased.

When we think of respect, it is a sense of worth or worthiness that is engendered (Dillon 1995). Mutual respect includes both self-respect and respect for others and from others. The idea of mutual respect points to the interactive, reciprocal nature of respect. For respectful interaction, we need to be able both to speak and be heard, and also to be able to listen. At times, an attitude of respect is not easily achieved, especially if our perspective is different from the other person's point of view. Mutual respect, however, is essential for real communication and 'communication with others is a part of the work of ethics itself' (Gustafson 1963, p. 18). The ethical question, 'How should I act?' is always raised within community. The response, therefore, needs to be found through dialogue, and in the interactions and relationships among patients, families, and professionals:

A relational ethics approach to K'aila's situation may

have opened the issues in a less confrontational, more helpful way. Respect can influence care situations so that patients and families experience less vulnerability when faced with the power of the medical system. It can change the process of choice-making from one that is autonomous to one that is shared, from one that separates people to one that connects them. A consultation with an ethics committee and more active support of conversations among parents, other family members, the physician and other caregivers might have maintained the relational aspects of K'aila's situation.

We need to cultivate a sensitivity to others that allows genuine dialogue. Both health care professionals and those they serve need the support of a climate of mutual respect.

The ethical demands of health care practice are far from simple. Like all ethical demands, they are 'abominably vague, confused and confusing' (Baumann 1993). Recognising this can help us. We will then be more willing to remain uncertain about our use of power, to look beyond professional agency and expertise, and to be open to other kinds of questions. Mutual respect, or the striving towards it, can in a constructive way shape our everyday encounters with pressing ethical dilemmas.

CONCLUSION

A relational ethic is an action ethic that has the potential to serve as a foundation for health care. The major claim of this approach is that ethical practice is situated in relationship and thus, knowing how to act and determining the right thing to do, must be developed within our relations with one another. This claim challenges any expectation that ethical knowledge can be secured once and for all or can be held as a type of expertise by a few knowledgeable sages. John Caputo (1989) has put it nicely:

We act not on the basis of unshakable grounds but in order to do what we can, taking what action as seems wise, and not without misgivings. We act, but we understand that we are not situated safely above the flux and that we do not have a view of the whole... We act because something has to be done (p. 59).

There is often no ethical certainty available in practice. We can, of course, ready ourselves as ethical professionals: learn the theories and principles of ethics; know the codes that our disciplines have set forth; be aware of paradigm cases; develop clinical expertise and communications skills; and cultivate the virtues that we admire. Most importantly, we must strive to be open to the ethical questions. We need to ensure that we do not lose ethical moments because we are insensitive to them. Staying open to the vulnerability and suffering of those in our care can be incredibly challenging. It is, however, the truly ethical thing to do.

REFERENCES

Anonymous 1985 Dax' case: who should decide? [video] Unicorn Media for Concern for Dying

Anonymous 1993 A choice for K'aila [video]. (Man Alive Series) Canadian Broadcasting Corporation, Ottawa

Austin W 2001 Nursing ethics in an era of globalization. Advances in Nursing Science 24 (2): 1–18

Baumann Z 1993 Postmodern ethics. Blackwell, Oxford

Beauchamp T L, Childress J F 2001 Principles of biomedical ethics, 5th edn. Oxford University Press, New York

Bergum V, Dossetor J (in press) Relational ethics: the full meaning of respect. University Publishing, Hagerstown, MD

Bhabha H K 1994 The location of culture. Routledge, London

Burt R, Cowart D 1998 Confronting death. Who chooses, who controls? Hastings Center Report 28 (1): 14–24

Caputo J D 1989 Disseminating originary ethics and the ethics of dissemination. In: Dallery A B, Scott C E (eds) The question of the other: essays in contemporary continental philosophy. State University of New York Press, Albany, NY, p. 55–62

Carper B A 1978 Fundamental patterns of knowing in nursing. Advances in Nursing Science 1 (1):13–23

Dillon R S 1992 Respect and care: toward moral integration. Canadian Journal of Philosophy 22 (1): 105–132

Dillon R (ed) 1995 Dignity, character, and self-respect. Routledge, New York

Duff R 1987 'Close-up' versus 'distant' ethics: deciding the care of infants with poor prognosis. Seminars in Perinatology 11 (3): 244–253

Gadow S 1999 Relational narratives: the postmodern turn in nursing ethics. Scholarly Inquiry for Nursing Practice 13 (1): 57–70

Gilligan C 1982 In a different voice: psychological theory and women's development. Harvard University Press, Cambridge, MA

Gustafson J M 1963 Introduction. In: Niebuhr H R The

responsible self. Harper and Row, New York

Kuhse H 1999 Some reflections on the problem of advance directives, personhood, and personal identity. Kennedy Institute of Ethics Journal 9 (4): 347–364

Levine M 1977 Nursing ethics and the ethical nurse. American Journal of Nursing 77 (5): 845–849

Løgstrup K 1956 The ethical demand (Jensen T trans 1971) Fortress Press, Philadelphia PA

Paulette L 1993 A choice for K'aila. Humane Medicine 9 (1): 13–17

Reynolds W, Scott P A, Austin W 2000 Nursing, empathy and the perception of the moral. Journal of Advanced Nursing 32 (1): 235–242

Schultz D, Carnevale F 1996 Engagement and suffering in responsible care giving: on overcoming maleficence in health care. Theoretical Medicine 17: 189–207

Smith D H 1992 Seeing and knowing dementia. In: Binstock R H, Post S G, Whilhouse P J (eds) Dementia and aging: ethics, values, and policy changes. Johns Hopkins University Press, Baltimore, MD, p. 44–54

Taylor C A 1993 Positioning subjects and objects: agency, narration and relationality. Hypatia 8 (1): 55–80

Veatch R 1998 The place of care in ethical theory. Journal of Medicine and Philosophy 23 (2): 210–224

Vetlesen A 1994 Perception, empathy and judgement: an inquiry into the preconditions of moral judgement. University of Pennsylvania Press, Pennsylvania. PA

6

Relational narratives: solving an ethical dilemma concerning an individual's insurance policy*

Robin Lindsay   Helen Graham

In this chapter Robin Lindsay and Helen Graham show how several different frameworks can combine to give one person the best possible care. Ethics, philosophy, nursing theory and professional working relationships are the 'ingredients' that helped to construct this chapter. Written within the American health care system, it focuses on the needs of one person, Justin, and the questions and answers that motivated the various parties to act not only rightly, but creatively. This chapter is a practical demonstration of the theory presented in the chapters on either side of it.

INTRODUCTION

Cardiac rehabilitation is a restorative process that attempts the physical reconditioning of patients after a cardiac event by means of a prescriptive exercise programme. The goals of the programme are individualized and the objective is to increase physical exercise tolerance over a period of 6–12 weeks. American insurance companies specify clearly which diagnoses qualify for reimbursement. Three diagnoses currently reimbursed for cardiac rehabilitation are recent myocardial infarction, stable angina and coronary bypass surgery. Justin, the subject of this article, did not fall into any of these categories. His diagnosis was cancer. The surgery being cardiac in nature, however, did necessitate the use of a heart–lung bypass machine. The fact that Justin's diagnosis was not heart related, but involved cardiovascular procedures, placed Justin in a financially precarious situation.

A discussion of feminist ethical theory is beyond the scope of this article, other than to acknowledge its impact on the shift away from traditional objective, rational, universal and paternalistic biomedical ethics as the only option in deciding ethical questions. The development of feminist theory has brought about an emphasis on personal experience as defined by the person living that experience, leading to the creation of a relational rather than rational ethics. Rational narratives specific to each individual situation are the tools by which relational ethics are expressed, and have been written about by several authors.[1-5] Two relational narratives are described in the story presented here. The primary narrative occurs between a cardiac rehabilitation nurse and an insurance representative. A relational narrative is also formed between Justin and the cardiac rehabilitation nurse. The relational narratives described in this story depict how an uncovered insurance benefit eventually becomes available to Justin through a process of deconstruction, a process of chipping away at an ensconced traditional insurance policy. Expressed in postmodern terms, what occurs is the deconstruction of Justin's pre-existing policy. The authors believe that there is a practical fit between Gadow's ethical framework and Keller's concept of relational autonomy that is clinically useful not only between patient and

* Reprinted from Nursing Ethics 2000; 7(2): 148-157, by kind permission of the publisher, Arnold, London.

nurse but between nurse and, in this case, insurance company. This article attempts to show how Keller extends Gadstow's work and this becomes a conceptual framework for Justin's story, an example of the creative use of rational narratives. We believe more will become evident as this framework is used in clinical settings.

THE STORY

Justin is a 28-year-old man, married, and a junior executive in Corporate America. He is also a marathon biker. After seeking medical advice for increasing 'shortness of breath' when biking, eventually, over a two-month period, he was diagnosed with a sarcoma that extended from the ascending aorta to the right atrium of the heart. The cancer had also metastasized to the lungs. Soon after the dreaded diagnosis he underwent surgery. His hospital recovery was uneventful, in the sense that he had no postoperative complications.

Several days after surgery, the cardiac rehabilitation staff received an order for cardiac teaching to include chest wound and sternal healing precautions. During the teaching, the cardiac rehabilitation nurse, Kathy, noted in his history that he had always been an avid exerciser. Kathy and Justin spent time exploring what was significant to him. During this relational narrative they discussed his activity and exercise regime after hospital discharge. The issue of Justin's participation in the outpatient cardiac rehabilitation exercise programme came up during the teaching. Justin and his wife Melissa were interested in the prospect that Justin would soon be able to return to exercising in a safe environment. A major obstacle was recognized early on: who would pay for the outpatient exercise programme since his diagnosis did not warrant rehabilitation? Outpatient rehabilitation programmes without insurance are costly, particularly if the individual has to pay themselves.

Justin decided to sign up one week after discharge, with the understanding that he may have to cancel the appointment if attempts at financial reimbursement were unsuccessful.

Justin's case would be the first attempt at trying to bring a patient without underlying heart disease into the cardiac rehabilitation programme. The staff were convinced that, based on the type of surgery carried out, he had a chance, although remote, of receiving the benefit. In previous years the staff had successfully rehabilitated several individuals with a diagnosis of heart disease who were concurrently undergoing chemotherapy. The cardiac rehabilitation staff were convinced that, given a chance, Justin could regain his strength sooner and begin to focus on the positive aspects of healing and health through his participation in this comprehensive inter-disciplinary exercise programme.

Next, Kathy began a dialogue about this dilemma with an insurance representative from Justin's health plan. Annie, the representative, checked the insurance policy manuals. Unfortunately she discovered that Justin's case did not fit into any of the guidelines under which cardiac rehabilitation would be covered. Given these circumstances, the dialogue between Kathy and Annie could easily have ended here; however, it did not. It was at this juncture that a relational narrative developed between the nurse and the insurance representative. The uniqueness of Justin's situation touched Kathy and Annie, and prompted them not to file the case away but to pursue seeking additional benefit for him. Together they engaged themselves in Justin's situation and became his advocates. Numerous phone calls between the nurse and the insurance representative ensued to make this happen. Letters of medical necessity followed the calls. At Annie's instigation, Justin's case was eventually taken before the insurance company's board of appeals. As a result, approval came from the medical director of the insurance company. Justin would receive not only some, but all, of the services provided by the cardiac rehabilitation programme.

Kathy, Justin's nurse, and Annie, the insurance representative, initially became involved in this situation as part of their routine responsibilities. They agreed that Justin's situation presented a dilemma and they pursued solutions. Had they accepted an insurance denial, they would have been responding from a modern, positivist perspective. Autonomy within a relational narrative – the ability to maintain self-respect and be fully engaged without losing one's self – guided their actions in a postmodern contextual way. This led them through a process of the deconstruction of a traditional insurance policy into a creative reconstruction, which allowed Justin to receive the benefits he clearly needed.

First efforts undertaken to obtain reimbursement for the exercise programme equated with the deconstruction of the policy. A shift from a positivist paradigm to a humanistic, relational paradigm occurred. Insurance policies are closely aligned to a modern paradigm that is 'structured, controlled, hierarchical'.[6]

In this story, subjective experiences have been extrapolated from real events. It is through these occurrences that postmodernism displaces a positivist ideology. A mutual understanding results from the relational narrative formed between the nurse and the insurance representative. The ensuing dialectic positioned Justin's advocates to consider all possibilities for recovery. Together, they deconstructed a pre-existing policy that had proved to be of no benefit to their patient. This concept can best be understood in the context of Justin's story by considering Bent's discussion of statements by Powers[7] and Reed[8] that 'all conceptual essences, even those of meaning and power, are rejected in favor of situated accounts,'[7] where either/or problems are not solved but deconstructed in the search for a practical significance'[8] (p. 80).[6] The extension of relational narrative by relational autonomy is one framework through which to accomplish this.

AN ETHICAL FRAMEWORK

'Ethics' can be a dreaded word. There is always someone who is not satisfied either with the answer or the process by which it is decided. Parts of the traditional biomedical system are based on authority, rules, certainty and final answers. In a fast-moving clinical setting the sheer impracticality of spending the time

haggling over points and tallying them up to make a final decision can drive practitioners back to the ward and the pressing work of patient care. A rationalist decision is made by the majority of a committee, who are often rational, modern thinkers. Yet, as Tisdale writes in *The sorcerer's apprentice* (p. 11–12),[5] one traditional ethics system 'is too small to contain the problem it hopes to solve. Ethics is the study of conduct and behavior, the study of response, antiphony, and echo. It is inherently fluid – fluid as in provisional.' This is a postmodern stance that is becoming increasingly familiar to nurses, and is clearly not authoritarian, objective or certain. In this stance there is no single solution for rational thinkers and no comfortable telos for relational thinkers. Each dilemma is absolutely unique; each behaviour evokes a provisional response; the narrative is fluid.

Justin's story demonstrates how a fluid conceptual framework can be created through combining two previously described intersubjective exchanges focusing on patient advocacy: Gadow's concept of the relational narrative[1,2] and Keller's concept of relational autonomy.[3] The following discussion shows how these two concepts can be extended into a learned skill that is practical in a nursing setting, as was shown in Justin's case.

In her most recent article, 'Relational narrative: the postmodern turn in nursing ethics',[2] Gadow recognizes three layers that are part of the ethical cornerstone of a philosophy of nursing (Table 6.1). The layers are identified as: subjective immersion, objective detachment, and relational narrative. (She has also identified these layers as premodern, modern and postmodern respectively. For the sake of clarity the first three terms will be used, although the reader is cautioned that the two sets of terms are sometimes used interchangeably because of their similar characteristics.) According to Gadow, subjective immersion is characterized by certainty because it is unreflective. It is based on moral tradition, religion or other source outside the self that is 'powerful enough to resist reflection' (p. 5). Its corresponding era, premodernism, yields no ethical questions

Table 6.1 Gadow's characteristics of philosophical layers

Layer	Nature of ethical dilemma
Premodern: subjective immersion Immersion in belief Myth, religion, family and community values No thought of doing things another way Unquestioning	No ethical dilemmas because there are no questions
Modern: objective detachment Rational, objective, empirical Authoritative, paternalistic Utilitarian, final answer sought Rigorous inquiry, systematic procedures Logical positivism, reductionistic All individual cases regarded equally	Ethical dilemma is stepped outside of and viewed objectively No more than one interpretation allowed
Postmodern: relational narrative Passionate engagement, relationship Co-authorship, narrative Situated perspective, safety Uncertainty embraced, no absolutes	Answers to ethical dilemmas are constructed and contingent and can be deconstructed according to changes in situation or interpretation

because the tradition provides both ethical appraisal of the situation and nursing action that is unarguable.

Detachment, the second layer, is also characterized by uncertainty in Gadow's view. It is a system of rational objectivity – 'one incontestable system of universal principles' (p. 7) – that respects individuals equally in all cases, paradoxically leaving little room for the vagaries of individuality. Distance is always maintained to provide objectivity and to avoid more than one interpretation of ethical questions. Its corresponding era, modernism, has been linked with such terms as logical positivism, reductionism, utilitarianism, universalism, authoritarianism, empiricism and paternalism. Although all individuals are respected equally, that very quality demands that the same principle be applied in every case (as in Justin's case before negotiations with the insurance company began). Gadow points out that there is less certainty in this layer than is at first apparent.

Interpretations of a principle can cause conflict in clinical settings; the application of a principle in some settings requires force; and universalism devalues the uncontrollable, as it did Justin's need for the emotional and physical benefits of cardiac rehabilitation although no coronary artery bypass operation was actually carried out.

Gadow's third layer, relational narrative – 'the words the nurse and patient compose together, the words of their engagement' (p. 10)[2] – yields ethical knowledge that is co-authored, contingent and contextual. This requires deep listening, a 'being there' that is sometimes thought to be self-sacrificing, but which in reality is mutual participation with specific guidelines for the nurse (which Keller provides). This layer corresponds to the postmodern era, which 'resists the modern drive for unity, order and foundations. Every form of order becomes a target for deconstruction' (p. 9)[2] from the social to the hermeneutic order. Meanings are assigned by individuals with no authoritative ground on which to stand, and are thus contingent on the ability to engage with another human being. Engagement between nurse and patient can yield a relational narrative that helps a patient to view a disability as a new ability, to assign an empowering meaning to an otherwise intolerably vulnerable circumstance (such as Justin's perceived loss of all his athletic ability). Because the dilemma can change, no answer is certain or final.

An understanding of Keller's model of relational autonomy broadens and clarifies Gadow's definition of the relational narrative of engagement and makes it easier to apply clinically. Keller places relational autonomy within the relational narrative as a responsibility of the practitioner.[3] Gadow alludes to relational narrative as a 'safer home, existentially, than would be found in subjective or objective certainty [which] would cost the nurse and patient their relationship' (p. 11).[2] Keller, building on Meyers[9] and Davion,[10] points out *how* relational narrative is a safer existential home using the concept of relational autonomy. In her article, 'Autonomy, relationality, and feminist ethics', Keller[3] defines relational autonomy in three parts: self-governance, being able critically to reflect on whether one can take responsibility for an action while being true to oneself; and the ability to learn and use this skill among friends and other social contacts (an intersubjective, relational exchange). Relational autonomy within a relational narrative allows the use of moral judgement in deciding what care to give and renders 'self-immolating care' (p. 159)[3] an argument against care ethics that is applicable only to those who deliberately choose it. Keller discusses Meyers' emphasis on relational autonomy as a learned skill. She suggests that a possible way to learn it is, when faced with an ethical dilemma, to picture a variety of solutions with a friend; imagine the results of carrying them out; and rely on feelings of self-respect for the decision chosen. The question to be answered is: 'Can I live with this?' The thoughtful integrity of the nurse on hearing the expressed desires of the patient (or physician or insurance company) becomes a carefully crafted synthesis between premodern, modern and postmodern ethical thought. The nurse learns to move with fluidity among layers of ethical thought while maintaining both autonomy and engagement by practicing Keller's steps. All taking part are potentially strengthened as the joint question becomes: 'Can we live with this?' This provides the fluid framework Tisdale (p. 11)[5] asks for, in which the patient and the practitioners of all layers of thinking may work in harmony – from unquestioning belief to objective empirical thought to authored, contingent and contextual engagement – and, through this intersubjectivity, provide a shared, and thus safer, existential home. Keller's steps were followed in Justin's case.

APPLICATION OF THE FRAMEWORK

Family, community belief system, tradition, religion and myths are a few examples associated with immersion, the first philosophical layer. Premodern immersion in Justin's story is depicted clearly through several characters. The extended family believed that the best medical treatment was available only from 'recognized' large medical centres. Thus, Justin's father pushed to have him treated elsewhere. The cardiovascular surgeon consented with hesitation to the outpatient exercise programme, stating: 'He doesn't have longer than six months but go ahead and give it to him if it makes him feel better.' Operating room and telemetry unit nurses treated the situation with dismal attitudes, leaving Justin and Melissa feeling isolated. Kathy also felt little support but was unable to let Justin go without a push for an insurance payment for the programme.

In Arthur Frank's autobiography, *At the will of the body*, he writes about his experience of living with cancer. He acknowledges how important it is for the medical and nursing staff to share emotions with patients who are experiencing terminal diagnoses. He writes: 'Anybody who wants to be a caregiver, particularly a professional, must not only have real support to offer but must also learn to convince the ill person that the support is there' (p. 70).[11] This example is a demand that caregivers should go beyond the stages of immersion and detachment to develop a relational narrative, and that the nurse is clear about her relational autonomy, her ability to maintain self-respect during an ethical dilemma.

Modern ethics is a move away from immersion to rational objectivity,[2] the second philosophical layer. Examples of detachment occur throughout this narrative. The chemotherapy treatment was one. Having critical decisions to make with regard to a treatment plan, Justin was flown to a large cancer centre institute, where 'state of the art' drugs were prescribed for chemotherapy. Although anxious to return home, he instead 'stuck it out', because this centre is the 'Mecca' for cancer treatment, but he never developed a relational, caring narrative with any caregiver there.

Beneficence, the assumption that the professional knows best, is a virtue associated with modern objectivity. The cardiac rehabilitation staff's claim that 'exercise will strengthen and improve your·health', to a degree demonstrates a paternalistic viewpoint. When Justin, Melissa and Kathy discussed Justin's choice to participate, his attitudes and opinions were finally taken into consideration, prompting a relational narrative to occur. A typical dialogue sounded like this:

Kathy: Good news! The insurance finally came through! Justin can participate in the entire programme!
Melissa: I don't know, Kathy. He might not be up to it any more. He's lost a lot of energy.
Kathy: No problem. That's what this programme is designed for. He'll build up strength in no time.
Melissa: (still doubtful) His strength is OK, if he would just get up. But he seems depressed to me…
Kathy: (finally addressing Justin) Justin, what do you think?

Lastly, the attitude of third party payers reflects a utilitarian attitude. Again a modern perspective is evident. What is best for the majority of individuals, with little harm to 'others' echoes the detachment of the insurance company in Justin's situation. This translates into: 'Although Justin may benefit from the programme, there are many other beneficiaries needing the resources that are covered benefits.' Whether they would be efficiently, effectively or even used at all did not take away their status as covered benefits. The challenge became, how could the cardiac rehabilitation centre provide the requested services when they were not part of his insurance package? In addition, a dearth of scientific knowledge proving that exercise would benefit Justin's condition served to limit further Justin's chances of receiving benefits.

THE RELATIONAL NARRATIVE IN POSTMODERN TERMS

Although an important relational narrative existed between Justin, Melissa and Kathy, it is not *the* narrative emphasized here. The actual narrative of focus is the dialogue that occurred between Kathy and the insurance agent. The refusal by the insurance company to reimburse a clearly necessary treatment because it was not in the plan was modern in nature. However Kathy and the insurance agent (acting with relational autonomy) did not see this reply as acceptable. A typical exchange would be:

Kathy: This man is so motivated; he's an athlete and used to physical exercise but afraid he'll never be able to do it again. I am afraid the normal postsurgical depression will deepen into a depression that could be averted with this therapy. His wife is very supportive. It won't be a waste of money. I can say that for sure.
Annie (insurance agent): Let me see if I can find some loopholes into which he fits. You know I can't just grant authority.
Kathy: Yes, I know. But you can see how it might be worth it for this man? It will be therapeutic in several ways. The exercise should help him to maintain his stamina throughout the chemotherapy. By giving Justin this therapy I believe we may see less depression and a better response to the chemotherapy.
Annie: Yes, I see. I can tell how much you care and how convinced you are. Let me see what I can do. It may not be anything, though, so don't get your hopes up.
Kathy: Thank you for your time! Hopefully there will be a way.

Together, Kathy and Annie's efforts and rallying behind a treatment plan that Justin desired is considered postmodern in nature. They believed that Justin would benefit in numerous ways. Based on several first-hand experiences Kathy had been involved with in the past, she had witnessed individuals who had been diagnosed with heart disease and cancer exercising in a supervised programme. She saw what appeared to be significant results

Table 6.2 Characteristics of a fluid model of nursing ethics

Ethical stance	Characteristics	Examples
Subjective immersion	No ethical question	Justin's extended family 'Your plan doesn't pay.'
Objective detachment	One interpretation of ethical question	'State of the art' drugs 'Exercise will help you'
Relational narrative	Answers to ethical question cocreated, contingent	Narrative between Kathy and Justin, Melissa and doctors
Relational autonomy within relational narrative	Responsibility of practitioner; fluid movement and synthesis between all ethical stances 'Can we live with this?' is the ethical question	Kathy's refusal to accept insurance limitations, which led to narrative involving family, doctors, insurance agent, insurance medical director, etc. Included but was not limited to ethical solutions from all stances above

concerning overall health status correlated with a structured exercise regimen. With participation in an exercise programme these individuals maintained muscle mass, strength and weight while undergoing chemotherapy. In the end, the efforts undertaken to obtain reimbursement for the exercise programme equated to the 'deconstruction' of an existing insurance policy.

The positive outcome of this story contradicts the popular conception of medical insurance companies as intransigently greedy. It is to be hoped that the weight of public opinion is beginning to have its effect on the medical insurance industry. Justin's story demonstrates the possibility that policies of wisely managed insurance companies can be deconstructed for the benefit of an individual.

Another layer of significance involves the potential role of the nurse in the future. It is clear from this story that nursing can play a major role in the planning and securing of health care benefits for patients through the use of autonomy within relational narratives. Other ethical decisions can

also be influenced by using the more flexible, fluid ethical model described here. Justin's story illustrates the dynamics of relational narratives involving several ethical decisions. Some should be considered before closing his story.

As mentioned earlier, Justin was a young corporate worker, productive and athletic. Would the pursuit of benefits have been as aggressive had Justin been unemployed, unpleasant or even physically unattractive? Furthermore, in a society where youth is regarded highly, consider the impact of a similar situation had the patient been an elderly individual. Some might ask, although the programme was desired by Justin, Melissa and also the cardiac rehabilitation staff, was it medically necessary for him? There is also the real question of whether, given the finite resources available and Justin's condition and prognosis, was cardiac rehabilitation cost-effective from the insurance company's perspective or even from the general perspective of allocating health care dollars wisely? The answers to these questions require the use of the addition of Keller's relational autonomy to Gadow's relational narrative to produce a compassionate and responsible engagement (Table 6.2).

THE ETHICAL FRAMEWORK REVIEWED

The authors have attempted to show how these, and countless other ethical questions, all unique and therefore impossible to fit into a single rational, objective formula, can be dealt with by the use of relational narratives and exchanges using both Gadow's and Keller's concepts. This was illustrated through the story of a real person. Because postmodern thought dictates that all individuals are unique and situated, the only way to know what they know is to hear their personal narratives, to 'walk in their souls', to 'compose together the words of their engagement' (p. 11).[2] Gadow affirms that a relational narrative seeks good for both parties; therefore, it is a relational ethic as well. Keller describes the 'wide latitude' a nurse has in deciding how to exercise her or his autonomy in participating in ethical questions (p. 160).[3] Far from being a contaminant of objectivity and moral certainty, autonomy within the relational narrative is critical in the ethical decision-making process, providing the subjective data that has been missing for so long. Keller puts the necessary restraint on the moral agents involved by insisting that autonomy and self-respect are mutually enhancing, whether alone or in a relational narrative, and are practised in the context of self-governance. Objective and subjective stances work together. Indeed, the simplicity of this framework is that, simultaneously, the preferred methods of all eras can flourish on the same hospital floor, with fluidity and in relative harmony. Justin's narrative, with all those who inhabit it, is a clear example of relational autonomy practiced within a relational narrative. This cohabitation need not be at the expense of the nurse, the patient or the ethics committee. Because no perfect answer is required, there is no deadline to meet. One must try responsibly to 'sing in perfect pitch with that individual patient's song, [for your] melody reaches God' (p. 119).[12]

ADDENDUM

Justin's managed care insurer could have denied his cardiac rehabilitation treatment. This would have been a safe corporate choice. Because of the relational narrative between the nurse and the insurer, a different course was taken. Justin is alive today, two years after the cardiac rehabilitation following surgery for sarcoma and his third course of chemotherapy. He has returned to full-time work and makes regular use of the outdoor pool and biking territory near his new home.

REFERENCES

1 Gadow S. Aging as death rehearsal: the oppressiveness of reason. J Clin Ethics 1996; 7: 335–40.
2 Gadow S. Relational narrative: the postmodern turn in nursing ethics. Schol Inquiry Nurs Pract 1999; 13: 3-16.
3 Keller J. Autonomy, rationality and feminist ethics. Hypatia 1997; 12: 152–165.
4 Parker R. Nurses' stories: the search for a relational ethic of care. Adv Nurs Sci 1990; 13(1): 31–40.
5 Tisdale S. The sorcerer's apprentice. New York: Henry Holt, 1986.
6 Bent K. Seeking the both/and of a nursing research proposal. Adv Nurs Sci 1999; 21(3): 76–89.
7 Powers P. Discourse analysis as methodology for nursing. Paper presented at the Fifth Annual Critical and Feminist Perspectives in Nursing Conference; 1994 Mar; Bothell (WA). Cited in: Bent K. Seeking the both/and of a nursing research proposal. Adv Nurs Sci 1999; 21(3): 76–89.
8 Reed PG. A treatise on nursing knowledge development for the 21st century: beyond postmodernism. Adv Nurs Sci 1995; 17(3): 70–84. Cited in: Bent K. Seeking the both/and of a nursing research proposal. Adv Nurs Sci 1999; 21(3): 76–89.
9 Meyers D. Personal autonomy and the paradox of feminine socialization. J Philos 1987; 84: 619–28.
10 Davion V. Autonomy, integrity, and care. Soc Theory Pract 1993; 19: 161–82.
11 Frank A. At the will of the body. Boston, MA: Houghton Mifflin, 1991.
12 Davis C. Poetry about patients: hearing the nurse's voice. J Med Humanities 1997; 18: 111–25.

7

Narrative ethics

Verena Tschudin

All the other authors have told stories to make their points. In this chapter, Verena Tschudin seeks to build an ethic on the premise that stories are fundamental to living and human flourishing. In starting with a story from the East, she weaves many aspects of this and other stories together to create the metastory of a narrative ethic, showing that dialogue, reflection and discussion lead to responsibility and action.

INTRODUCTION

Perhaps the most important word in English is 'and'. Everything in life starts with 'and' because there is always something that went before, and everything continues because history never ends. Thus every story really begins with 'and'. It is the word that binds people with people, and people with their experiences and surroundings. Not only do we make and tell stories, but stories also create who we are; thus, in telling stories we have to be aware that there is always more to what is spoken and heard, and that the story goes on long after it is 'finished'. The stories that individuals tell also create a bigger story: the metastory of a nurse and a patient, of families, of cultures.

This chapter is about stories, so I will first tell a story.

Monkey, or Sun Wu-K'ung in Chinese, was a clever and resourceful creature. He carried a magic stick and was riding a magic cloud. He defied the authorities of the heavens by eating the peaches of eternal life, but was brought to heel by the Buddha and imprisoned under a

stone mountain for 500 years. On his release he helped a monk, Tripitaka, who was on a journey from China to India, to search for sacred scriptures. Accompanying them were the pig monster, Pigsy, and the sand-eel monster, Sandy. Pigsy, or Zhu Bajie, was strong and had once got drunk and misbehaved with the Goddess of the Moon. He was punished by being sent to earth. Mystical Sandy, Sha Heshang, was a disgraced soldier of the Jade Emperor's army, who was sent to earth as a hideous monster, where the Emperor of heaven continued to torment him. Out of hunger he was driven to kill and eat travellers that passed by. When he was found by Tripitaka, he was no longer punished and he became a priest. By now the four travelled together and their journey was full of incidents and accidents, but Monkey continually pushed them on with his energy, colour, antics, mischief, magic, and acrobatic delights and infuriation. The journey led to rivers that were too wide and mountains that were too high, but they went on, searching not only for the holy scriptures that speak about enlightenment, but for enlightenment itself.

There is more to this story than might at first have appeared to the person who saw the Pantomime 'Monkey!' (written by Colin Teevan, directed by Mick Gordon) at the Young Vic Theatre in London in the 2001/2002 season (C Teevan, unpublished programme notes, 2001).

The monk Tripitaka is a historical figure from the seventh century CE. He brought the Sutra back with him from India to China and translated them into Chinese, thus effectively standardising Buddhist teachings there. Tripitaka means 'three baskets', because the scriptures are in three parts, originally written on palm leaves and preserved in baskets (Metz 1988). Monkey is a god and a king, but he is also a popular folk hero. Monkeys are noisy animals, up and down trees, fun to watch and be with, and all of us know the restless and unstable 'monkey mind' that gave this character his attributes. In the monkey we meet the childish mind: egoistical and demanding. As people grow they encounter the soul in the form of the monk Tripitaka, the appetites as Pigsy, and the intuition as Sandy. These characters are on the journey of humankind: they are 'Everyman' and 'Everywoman'. We are all on a journey. The journey is forward, but at some time we also have to return and come home, as if to our own self. This is perhaps the longest journey we undertake; we cannot avoid it. Illness or disaster often thrust us on a journey that we might never have wanted to make and do not know where it will lead us, but journey we must. It is the story of the journey that we need to tell and share and hear for the story to become 'real'.

NARRATIVE AS ETHICS

Not every story is an ethical story. It is in how the story is told, or why, that it becomes an ethical story. A person who says, 'a bird came and sat on my window sill' is stating a fact. If that person lives alone and has not spoken to anyone for a week, then the bird may have been his or her only companion. If the person is telling a friend about the bird as part of a longer story, perhaps relating it to incidents as a child or her work, then there is a much wider meaning in the telling of a simple fact. If the bird is unusual or exotic, it may have escaped, and thus it may certainly be an ethical story. In telling and hearing about a bird, two people are creating a new story, and this may become the metastory: the 'and'.

For the 50th anniversary of the NHS, Becky Maltby and Stephen Pattison (1999) published a collection of stories told to them by patients and staff: 'chief executives, nurses, doctors, administrative and clerical staff, health authority managers, health care assistants and a chaplain' (p. 1). They wanted to hear what values prevail in the NHS. The stories are simply retold, but not analysed specifically. In their general summing up, the authors write:

Stories offer us a way in to seeing living values or values in action. A story calls upon us to identify with it, and this process changes us by prompting us to re-interpret our views, to rethink the impact of our action. Whilst our response to a story tells us something about ourselves, sharing our responses moves us beyond where we are (p. 41).

In similar vein, Robert Veatch (1979) writes that 'medical ethics becomes interesting and relevant only when it abandons the ephemeral realm of theory and abstract speculations and gets down to practical questions raised by real, everyday problems of health and illness … It is real-life, flesh-and-blood cases which raise fundamental questions' (p. 1).

Ethics makes sense when we engage with it. It is in hearing other people's stories—their values, beliefs, reasons and reasoning, whys and wherefores—that we can engage with these things ourselves. Stories are therefore essential elements to learning about ethics and learning to be ethical beings. We have to hear other people's stories and we have to tell our own stories. Each story has to be told and heard. Stories have the capacity to be reflected upon and to change individuals and societies.

Postmodernism has left us with few certainties. We have largely lost the 'stories'—or even 'a' story—by which individuals, families and communities used to live. These were the stories about justice, human dignity, and what 'collectivity' meant. They were about honour, hope, direction and how and where to channel desire (Thomasset 1996). In order to know how to access these values and to create the ethical desire, we have to make our own story or stories. Sally Gadow has written widely about narratives within ethics. Her most detailed theory (Gadow 1999) considers three ages or types of ethics. In premodern ethics the family, tradition and community were the main elements, giving a subjective certainty. In modern ethics the outstanding elements are principles, theories and codes, leading to an objective certainty. In postmodern ethics there is an intersubjective contingency based on relational narrative. The postmodern idiom is essentially existentialist, stressing the uniqueness of the individual. However, individuals are also relational beings. Our relationships are close and real and utterly necessary, but they are not necessarily the same kind as those of earlier generations. Fifty years ago, our forebears often knew no one outside of their village or country; today we may know very few neighbours but have friends all over the world.

For an ethical theory or argument to make sense, it needs to lead to something: a decision, a way of working or being. It must be capable of transformation. In the words of Alain Thomasset (1996), 'only a narrative permits the establishment of a solid link between an action and a person who can be held responsible for it' (p. 171). A narrative (a story) is the link from theory to action. In reflecting on a story, there is also the movement from action to theory. Reflection is not simply a mode of learning or explanation, but a vital aspect of ethical thought and action.

In the postmodern idiom there are no superiors and inferiors but all are equal. It is therefore much more difficult to envisage that only one person would tell a story and only one other person would listen to it. Two people in any relationship are equal (they are ethically equal even if they are not socially equal) and therefore both need to tell their stories. They may be very different stories, and told for very different reasons, but the point is that the two people need to acknowledge their equal worth for an ethical relationship to exist and work. The distinction between expert and lay person is not acceptable. Both are experts, although perhaps in different areas. In living and telling the story about their lives, each is an expert, even though one of them may be a gifted story-teller and more like Monkey, and the other may be a person of few words and more like the monk Tripitaka. What one person says affects the other. What one lives affects the other. What patients say affects nurses. What nurses experience affects patients. In the nurse–patient dyad, each one's story is the means of enhancing the other and helping the other. It is not the quantity or literacy of the words spoken that matters, but *that* they are spoken, or enabled to be spoken. Caring may mean that nurses hear more stories from their patients than they tell them. *How* they hear these stories matters, and *what* they hear and do with what they hear, is crucial. This is the essence that makes the narrative to become an ethical narrative. 'Developing a narrative is a work of interpretation' (Thomasset 1996, p. 171).

HEARING THE ETHICAL NARRATIVE

Many people have written eloquently about caring for and listening to the other person. Perhaps no one has written more profoundly and poetically about 'the other' than Martin Buber in his *I and Thou* (1937). The relationships he describes can be used equally of other people as of a deity. At the deepest level, there is no distinction because we touch the spiritual and even the mystical when we touch the essence of relationships. When one is able to say 'Thou' within as well as to others, one truly relates to all that is present. It is therefore not surprising that Buber learned the hard way, epsecially the need to listen to oneself and the other so as to be present to the other. Marc Ellis (1997) writes:

Buber discovered this sense of presence in his early years as a professor in Germany. One afternoon, as often happened, a young man came to him asking for guidance. Buber, who spent extensive time in prayer, emerged from a morning of religious meditation and listened to the young man query him about the meaning of life. Buber conversed intently with him, yet in learning of the man's death a short while after their meeting, understood that he missed the essential content of the man's questions. Although Buber had been there in his physical being, because he was dwelling in the beauty of his religious enthusiasm, he was not fully present to the man's concerns. 'I learned that he had come to me not casually, but borne by destiny, not for a chat but for a decision,' Buber relates. 'He had come to me, he had come in this hour. What do you expect when we are in despair and yet go to a man? Surely a presence by means of which we are told that nevertheless there is meaning.' From that moment on Buber gave up the idea of religious experience as being one of exaltation and ecstasy separated from the world and humanity. Rather, the religious became a sense of fullness of claim and responsibility to each other in the everyday events of life' (p. 154).

It is not necessarily the words said or exchanged that matter, but *how* we hear what is said, and what we listen for. One of the first principles for any would-be counsellor is to be there in body and mind, or 'wherever you are, be there'. Clearly this is easier said than done. Every nurse knows the situation of being in the middle of doing three things when a patient calls and asks: 'Tell me, am I going to get better or not?' Which of the four jobs—and people—now have priority? Making an appointment and saving one's agony until later may not be possible. Answering the last person with an 'of course, you are' may not be an option either.

It is essentially only possible to hear what any person's story is about if we ask or consider what the point of telling it is. Most of the time, as hearers, we should not answer this ourselves, thereby making assumptions, but we should ask the person herself or himself. By asking the person even the simplest question, we give that person the assurance that she or he matters, that we are interested in hearing the story, that we want to be open to what we hear and that we are willing to 'be there' for the time being. Some stories take only five minutes. Some stories are without words, but call for empathy (suffering-in) and sympathy (suffering-with) expressed entirely in presence.

Instead of making assumptions, it is not only more polite but also ethically respectful and more fitting, to ask what is happening to the person. The much more difficult but also crucial question is about meaning. What does the person mean by a certain word, expression, or phrase? What is the meaning of *this* being said at *this* moment, to *this* person, in *this* way? When we ask for the meaning we get to the core of a person's being or action. It is the question that Buber did not ask of his student. Buber was concerned with his own meaning and therefore missed the essential.

Asking for the meaning of a person's story is not an easy question; nor should it be done lightly. Only when we are prepared to stay and hear the answer should we ask for the meaning. Being willing to hear the answer means being willing to be challenged by what we hear, and that is the ethical nub because that essentially means that we have to reflect on what we hear and what we do with what we hear.

Nurses hear other people's stories, but their own are equally important and need to be heard. It is safe to say that most nurses live with some story equivalent to Buber's: in a moment of inattention something went wrong; a patient was left suffering because we did not care enough; perhaps a patient died because of something we did or omitted to do. It may be something that nobody else is aware of but we cannot forget it even if most of the time we do not think about it. Whatever it is, our own story will have affected us deeply and coloured the way we behave. Such incidents challenge our integrity, our values, and hence our ethics. Stan van Hooft (1995) argues that 'a life as lived will integrate demands within itself which, if followed, will secure the integrity and wholeness of that life' (p. 143). Therefore 'the minimal requirement for any morality ... is a teleology of human aspirations ... such a teleology must be grounded ... in the biography of individuals and cultures' (p. 144). We live with our stories, whatever they are, and, in order to make sense of them, we have to accept them into our lives, reflect on them and live with them. When the stories are about our own mortality, then we may have a new challenge and often need the reflection that another person can offer, so that this story, too, can become integrated into our lives. It is small wonder that nurses are often exposed to questions about life and death because they live and work with life and death all day.

Talking with patients, clients and their families and friends is not easy and, to avoid it, nurses often blame a lack of time. What tends to be forgotten is that it takes little time to engage with someone at a very deep and intimate level.

Spending a few minutes now with an anxious person may save hours later with a super-anxious person. Engaging on a personal level now with someone may also save treatments, medications, and perhaps even legal costs, later. Respecting a person for who she or he is, hearing what she or he is about and acknowledging this, is not only a far more humane way, it is also a more ethical way of dealing with a need.

In the same way, nurses are well aware of the fact that patients and clients often engage housekeeping personnel or technicians in talking about their needs. These members of staff have a more distant relationship and they may therefore be 'safer' than nurses and doctors who are aware of diagnoses and prognoses. The 'witness' role of many staff members is vital. Patients may be able to 'try out' on them how far they can go with questions. If such persons are aware of their role of witness, they can be invaluable, simply in giving assurance that the patient has been heard and the story has not been dismissed. Nurses sometimes resent that patients choose other staff than themselves with whom to share stories. Such resentment or envy is misplaced because we do not normally know the reasons why patients choose this person rather than another, and it is none of our business. What is far more important is that all personnel are able to help when and where appropriate, with respect and confidentiality. Thus the ethical standard of the institution is also raised, not only that of the individual.

What we hear in our own and other people's stories is uncertainty, insecurity, vulnerability, pain and fear. If everybody knew how to deal with these things, we would not be exposed to them. When we do not know how to handle a situation, we may be confused about which ethical principle applies: is truth the driving force, or doing good; is it a matter of duty or freedom; is it a right versus conscience; or is it loyalty versus duty? The person's moral code may suddenly have collapsed and long-held values become questionable. Such a person is truly disorientated. Telling the story of what is happening is therefore the only way to make some sense and re-orientate oneself. The story

needs to be told to another person; a brick wall will not do. This is why a relationship is important. The two people together create the ethics from the story told, heard, and responded to. What the outcome is cannot be envisaged or forced. The outcome—the telos—is what is fitting in each unique situation, although it is based on what has gone before ('and') in terms of personal, communal and social experience, and the outcome will also affect the person, the community and society. Michael Hardey (2002) describes the 'home pages' on the Internet that have been constructed by many people to write about the stories of their illness. This can also be taken metaphorically: the story told on a home page can lead to a new ethical understanding of one's life and illness, and therefore a 'home page' is the new understanding thus achieved when the story has been told in terms of ethics.

Nurses and patients may not necessarily exchange their stories, but it can help. The nurse who was talking about her own marital problems while showering a patient helped the patient to recognise a sense of usefulness in an otherwise useless existence (Tschudin 1995, p. 100–101). The nurse who said to a patient, 'if you think you have problems, just listen to mine', dismissed the patient's story because she could hear only her own. Had she heard the patient's story, they might have found much in common and been able to help each other. *What* we hear and how we hear it matters. This is a nursing skill as much as giving any treatment is, but it takes a personal commitment that cannot be demanded by either patients or employers. It demands the ethical commitment that stems from the person's own values and sense of responsibility.

THE ETHICAL METASTORY

A relationship is not simply to have someone to chat to, or to feel good in their presence. This may happen spontaneously, but what the relationship creates is what matters. When someone, such as a patient, tells a story, however short, to a nurse, this nurse and patient together create a bigger story, however limited. This metastory enables the listening, reflection, challenge, and perhaps re-ordering of values and beliefs that are called for and which will constitute the telos. Thus the relationship is vital to any kind of caring. The relationship is the basis and it is the vehicle for ethics to be done.

When a patient is not able to tell his or her story, or is silenced, paternalism is evident. When the nurses' voice is silenced by focusing only on the patient, Gadow (1996) calls this 'consumerism' (p. 8). When patient and nurse 'interpret their co-authored narrative, describing the good they are seeking' (p. 8), their narrative is no longer either general or personal, neither public nor private, but relational. Similarly, Gadow (1999) writes that in those moments when nurses glimpse

the abyss through a patient's eyes ... ethical certainties fail, and nothing remains except possible engagement between nurse and patient; but engagement is enough (without it a patient is alone, no matter how many nurses are present). The ethical narrative a nurse and patient compose through their engagement interprets the situation, saving it, for the moment, from meaninglessness (p. 64).

The nurse does not need to invoke theories and impress the patient with clever words. On the contrary, the simple words of everyday language are often more powerful and realistic to understanding what is happening. What happens in the body, soul, mind, memory or psyche is often confused and confusing, and can therefore be expressed only in simple words or images. These need to be captured and held in the present so that they can form the basis for building the wider and bigger story on them.

One of the very basic understandings of all interaction is that we constantly respond to what is said. Every response is made on the basis of what has been said or non-verbally conveyed and interpreted. Therefore, all people in any interaction are equally important. It is in this response to each other that we convey our humanity most. Because of how we respond, and through the ability we have to respond, we learn our responsibility. How we deal with each other in any setting shows us and others how willing we are to be responsible. In dialogue we

get to know each other and ourselves. Part of the responsibility is that we are willing to listen to and hear what others say, and also that they respond to what they hear from us. The one prerequisite for this is that we accept what every person says as valid without prejudice. Only in this way are persons fostered and not diminished. This does not preclude critical appraisal, but criticism also is made and given with respect for the person. These reasons and experiences have helped in understanding that ethics is learned in engaging in reflection and dialogue. If this dialogue be with a sick person or with a group of colleagues or students, it is this discussion, reflection and dialogue that constitutes the metastory. This becomes 'our' story and out of this come decisions and actions.

In postmodernism, where there are rarely any rules strong enough to guide individuals or groups, narrative becomes the main tool for working. Therefore, how the story is created is vital and must be learned. The really important narratives are about the suffering and loss experienced by everybody. When a story cannot be told because there is too much pain, it can sometimes be released simply by an embrace or even just by being present. Many people find that, when they are bereaved, they have to tell their story again and again, and, in the telling, some small item changes, indicating movement. We need to encourage each other to tell our stories. By telling a story we anchor an experience and give it a context. If a story is not told, we may forget it, and thus we may make some mistake again. This is particularly true of the big stories of our times: it is necessary to repeat the story of the Shoah (Holocaust) and the events of 11 September 2001 in America again and again, in order to be more acutely aware of the signs of any similar atrocities and to act to prevent them. As nations and societies we may not have been particularly successful in doing this, but at least we try to be ethically attentive. This demands that we *want* to listen and hear, and to acknowledge what was heard. It makes us sensitive to the terrorist and the Nazi within, for we are part of humanity and as such cannot not be involved or understand.

The metastory leads to compassion, if we enable it. This is a compassion that stops us from being victims or perpetrators, or bystanders. It demands that we become involved with ourselves and with others.

WHAT WE DO WITH THE ETHICAL NARRATIVE

We do not hear a story only to dismiss it or forget it. The poet John Donne (1624) stated that 'any man's death diminishes me, because I am involved in mankind', but more positively it would also be possible to say that 'any man's life enriches me, because I am involved in mankind'. Maybe today it would be more acceptable to say that 'whatever happens to anyone else also happens to me, because I am part of humanity'; or even, as Simone Roach (2002) suggests, we actually need the new kind of story that encompasses the universe as a community in bondedness, not bondage. Such a story is able to celebrate the earth as subject rather than as an object to be exploited and consumed. It also empowers people to see each other as participants rather than as observers, and as people who are engaged in a web of relationships where scientific relationalism is no longer possible.

Stories are told in relationships; people are in relationships. Neither people nor their stories exist in the abstract. Perhaps one of the really important things that is being learned in ethics at this time is that, unless we know how to be ethical beings and practice ethically, any theory of ethics is of little use. In nursing, as in many other disciplines, we have tended to start with the theory and then move into practice. Narratives teach us that the practice—the lived experience—comes first, and that only in reflection on the practice can we reach some theory. In telling each other our stories we are participants of all that happens, because we belong to each other. It is this commonality that emerges when the metastory is being constructed. It is then the commonality that leads to ethical action.

A number of themes have emerged when nurses have researched what happens in practice when stories of patients and nurses have been told:

- The need to keep the narrative going in order to stay focused
- Becoming aware of a personal moral commitment
- Becoming morally reflective
- Learning to live with ambiguity
- Nurturing community
- Creation of an atmosphere in which truth becomes discernible
- The emergence of the good within nursing
- Becoming aware of the lack of autonomy
- Becoming politically aware.

Keeping the narrative going

In order to stay focused, an individual 'must continually integrate events that occur in the external world and sort them into the ongoing "story" about the self' (Glen 1999, p. 7). Without clear social, civil and historical guidelines of ethical behaviour, individuals increasingly have to craft their own stories, simply in order to make sense of life. It is important to know where we have come from and how we have reached today, and, so that tomorrow makes sense, we have to understand our today. People who drift without reflection tend to become pathologically disillusioned or depressed. Being able to tell one's story, reflect on it with others so that it has a context and a purpose, and so that the good and the bad, positive and negative, the gains and the losses, can be integrated; all these are not only important but are part of being and becoming human.

The stories about the NHS that Maltby and Pattison (1999) collected were part of this process. They were surprised when they heard the stories, because they were aware that the NHS

subscribes to the values of equality of access, putting patient needs first, being caring, and valuing individuals and their differences. We found that it seems to be caught in a high level *debate about* its values, whilst *denying, ignoring, or just missing the reality* (emphasis added) of the values being lived out in day-to-day practice (p. 2).

It is this dichotomy that is brought to light in stories. Stories are about the real experience, while a debate can go into the stratosphere with wishful thinking. In the end it is the lived experience that is encountered, not the theory. Therefore the story has to continue so that the debate can become a narrative again.

Becoming aware of a personal moral commitment

In a study by Elisabet Sjöstedt and colleagues (2001), nurses were taught the importance of carefully managing the first nurse–patient encounter in a psychiatric setting by means of a conceptual model. The first encounter 'is of moral significance because the way in which nurses meet patients communicates the extent of their understanding of patients' vulnerability' (p. 313). When the nurses used the concepts of the model they had been taught, they were able to focus 'on their responsibility to encourage the patient to enter into a therapeutic relationship' (p. 317). Nurses were able to hear the patients' suffering and receive and contain strong emotions, and were able to help patients to feel less ashamed of being mentally ill. Patients and nurses were more involved in the overall care, and relationships were created in which the patients' sense of confidence and hope was encouraged. It meant that patients and nurses got to know and trust each other quickly, and this trust was sustained throughout the patients' stay. The nurses learned what a moral commitment in caring amounts to, and, having experienced this, they could trust the reality and feel more secure in this commitment.

Although these authors described an experiment that had to be stopped because of lack of funding, the fact that the authors told their story (in writing) shows that it entailed more than a good idea. Care is costly, both in terms of money and emotional involvement. The sad fact is that, too often, short-term expediency is preferred to long-term health. Perhaps this story needs to be told and experienced again and

again before it is 'heard' in the place or by the people who can actually make it happen. This is the kind of nursing that most nurses would prefer to engage in, leaving them more satisfied and the patients more respected, less anxious, more responsible, and thus perhaps less dependent on medication and institutions.

Becoming morally reflective

The same nurses (Sjösted et al 2001) reflected on their experience of this time of increased attention to the first nurse–patient encounter. They were made aware of the need to be flexible when dealing with patients. Although they followed a model, not all aspects of the model applied to all patients. They needed to be aware, at the moment itself, of some questions that could apply to individual patients and that some might not. The nurses became flexible and able to account for not asking certain questions in order not to invade a patient's privacy. They had also become more critical of their own and their colleagues' care when it was not the best possible. 'They tried to understand why their behaviour towards patients sometimes became opposite to what they intended' (p. 319). When a nurse 'really' met a patient in the first encounter, this 'inspired a feeling of self-confidence in the nurse and gave rise to both the patient's and the nurse's own hope of personal growth' (p. 319). This encounter, and the story the patient tells the nurse and that the nurse hears, and the metastory that the two created together, left everyone feeling good. For the nurses this meant 'being able to offer patients something more, based on nursing knowledge' (p. 319). This, after all, is what education in nursing knowledge is about.

Learning to live with ambiguity

A Scandinavian colleague of Sjöstedt, Eli Haugen Bunch (2001), observed life in a critical care unit in Norway. There were many obvious dramas taking place but, underneath the visible ones, Haugen Bunch found others emerging, which were less clear-cut and not always with a solution. She found that nurses were constantly concerned that the 'primary aim is the human being in the bed and not the machines. The machines must never dominate, they are helpful tools, we must provide care to a human being' (p. 63). This meant that every situation that could not be dealt with immediately took on an ethical dimension. The main dilemmas therefore were: end-of-life issues; patients who were transferred too soon to other hospitals; limited resources, leading to questioning if there should be an age limit for some types of surgery; limited resource allocations; and staffing levels. The team working there constantly discussed problems together. They considered if treatment should be continued for certain patients, but they never used cost to argue such a decision. Nurses and doctors would talk 'about treatment options, possible outcomes and what to do in case the patient required resuscitation' (p. 65). 'Decisions to terminate treatment were never made without the health providers and family attaining a consensus' (p. 66). These discussions engendered trust among all staff members, and thus the 'hidden' dramas were dealt with openly. 'The characteristics of the drama, plus uncertainty and ambiguity, are detailed in team conferences and discussed in an environment of openness and respect' (p. 66). When a patient's condition becomes uncertain, ambiguity necessarily follows. By talking together—creating their story—the team in this unit learned how to live with ambiguity rather than closure, contingency rather than closure, the emerging drama rather than the expected one. In this way they learned to be humane, to treat the human being rather than rely on machines. In this way they lived their experience by constantly re-telling and re-shaping their story.

Nurturing community

The physicist and systems theorist Fritjof Capra described (1998) how networking is common to all life forms. Not all networks are living systems, but 'one of the most important features of all living networks is that they involve feedback loops'. Hence, 'one of the best ways to nurture [a] community is to facilitate and sustain conversations' (p. 46). If plants and animals depend on their feedback loops, how much more important is it for members of any family, team or institution to hear what the others are saying and to act on this.

Capra talks of two different types of structures—designed and emergent—and believes that every organisation needs both kinds. Designed structures cannot grow, but they give stability. Emergent structures 'express the community's collective creativity' (p. 47). These structures are headed by different types of leadership. The designed-structure leader is a person who can formulate its mission, sustain this, and communicate well. Emergent-structure leadership is not limited to a single individual but can be distributed, because this depends on:

continually facilitating the emergence of new structures and incorporating the best of them into the organization's design. How does one facilitate emergence? By creating a learning culture, by encouraging continual questioning and by rewarding innovation. In other words, by creating conditions rather than giving directions. Facilitating emergence means nurturing a network of conversations (p. 47).

This analysis from physics echoes what Haugen Bunch found in the critical care unit whose staff constantly talked about the emergent situations. Thus they could work with the ambiguity of their patients' illness and decide on the needs of the person rather than on any policies or directives. Staff and families could therefore trust each other and work with each other. Nurturing the community is therefore a basic human need: the relationships count and these are maintained by the story they create together.

An atmosphere in which truth becomes discernible is created

In order to describe the essence of narrative, Sally Gadow (1995) compares nursing to a landscape. We can have a map of the land, but this is very different from actually being there. Experienced nurses are familiar with all the different aspects of their part of the land, and their job is to engage with and help to negotiate safe passage through this landscape for the people who find themselves there because of illness. Every country has different characteristics, which are sources of both strength and frailty. The people who live there know the vagaries of ice in the Arctic, and the wind, rain and tides in Britain. These vagaries can be conveyed only 'as narratives of exploration' (p. 213). Any situation that divorces people from their experience presents a dualism. 'In dualism the lived truth of experience remains elusive, whereas narrative creates an atmosphere in which truth becomes discernible' (p. 213). Telling our stories makes us subjects and authors of our own experiences. Thus, when others hear our stories, they can relate to the whole person, rather than to objects. When we treat others as objects, we hear only a small amount of the truth about them; the rest remains hidden because objects are looked *at*, whereas those who are subjects together look *with* each other. Looking together enables each other to discern and see the truth of each other. The more we talk, the more truth we encounter, about the other, about ourselves, and about the wider society.

All nurses know the damage that can be done when truth is hidden or suppressed. So that this damage can be eliminated, talking, discussing, reflecting, listening and hearing are necessary. No wonder that ethics is learned best in discussion, conversation and dialogue. This also clearly shows that it is not always a question of 'what' is truth, but 'when' is truth. It is not the quantity of truth, but the understanding of it. It is in this context that the word 'and' is often important, because, in health care, truth often emerges rather than exists as an object.

The emergence of the good within nursing

Cross-cultural studies of nursing activities can reveal similarities and differences in working that are surprising and unexpected. One such study, conducted by Dawn Doutrich and colleagues (2001) of nursing situations in the USA and Japan, found that theoretical and principle-based approaches to ethics had little relevance to daily patient care. Yet the stories they collected from the nurses they interviewed often showed an exquisite attuning of nurses to the needs of their patients. This was particularly evident for nurses in Japan, where the culture demands that nurses 'see behind the words' (p. 453) and respond to what they 'see'. The nurses did not use ethical language, but when the researchers analysed the stories told to them, 'the ethics seemed to come out of the practice and were centred on the particular patient in the particular situation'. Through these 'narratives, nurses express strong values and notions that surely relate to the good that is inherent in the profession'. The narratives 'were focused on involvement, communication, relationship and context' (p. 456) and from within a framework that matched the patients' needs. When nurses are able and enabled to give appropriate care, they know well how to do it. They also know how to put it into words in the stories they tell, and they do not need to use theoretical language to express what matters to them.

Becoming aware of the lack of autonomy

When nurses are aware of what they can and could do, they also become aware of what they cannot do. The reasons why their vision and practice are often limited are too numerous to mention. Nursing is often an 'in between' role: in between 'the physician's plan of medical care, the institution's policies and resources, and the patient's view of the good life' (Doutrich et al 2001, p. 456). This is not necessarily a bridging role, combining different aspects in the care given, but it is a buffer-role, keeping one side at bay against another. This takes an enormous amount of energy and leaves no side satisfied. It tends to be a warring stance because the kind of practice that is most suited to nursing is an emergent structure, which almost inevitably clashes with the designed structures of the institution's goals, the physician's medical model, and the patient's expectations. When they can be met, as Haugen Bunch (2001) described, it shows the strengths of all the structures. When this is not possible, unethical practice is too easily the reality. Defending one's corner, refusing to get involved in working relationships and practices, not reporting drug errors, abusing patients and colleagues, are all issues that tend to receive media attention. They can be seen as the outworkings of frustrations with systems that hinder creativity. If institutions and organisations demand ethical practice of their employees, they also have to act ethically towards them. The awareness of limited autonomy is not something that has to be accepted in a 'grin and bear it' mode, but something that has to be negotiated and worked through, therefore demanding listening and hearing.

Becoming politically aware

In describing the skills needed by nurses who work in commissioning in the health services, Sue Antrobus (2000) mentions four specific skills that are necessary if nurses are to be successful in influencing policy makers. In the light of this chapter, these skills are not at all limited to commissioning.

- Nurses need to show a much broader political awareness. They 'need to understand the direction of public policy in relation to public health' (Antrobus 2000, p. 39). In terms of this chapter, this is one of the by-products of ethical awareness. Having listened to patients and clients and their stories, nurses are challenged to be advocates; in this way they become politically aware, that is, knowing who to approach for action, and how. They cannot help but come to know the political situation and the players that influence them.
- Nurses need to identify the necessary leadership skills. Because they know what patients need and value, nurses need to transport these needs and values into the political arena, in which there is increasing interest in local and personal care, or at least 'people-focused' care. If nurses are able to identify and work with both designed and emergent leadership structures, they are also

able to work ethically, because such skills depend on hearing stories and working with them.

- Nurses need language skills. Because they are versed in several 'languages' (i.e. the languages of patients, medicine, counselling and therapy, humour, and that of any specialty in which they work) nurses are already highly skilled. They need to 'interpret' for the various parties or interested bodies. The skill of language is highly adaptive, involving moving between 'languages' and ensuring that all parties are understood. This demands a high level of listening skill and awareness.
- Nurses need to go beyond the restrictions of their status and boundaries. In an ethic where narratives are the basic tool, everyone is equal. This equality is an important aspect to acknowledge and maintain. In any political climate, the dominant parties look after their own, keen to maintain their designed structures. With their skills, nurses are able to put a different strategy alongside this and show that emergent strategies are also necessary, especially in the care of people. If patients matter, then so do nurses. Ethically, this is the only fitting way forward.

CONCLUDING REMARKS

Ethics is increasingly seen to be learned in discussion and reflection. Personal stories, not simply 'cases', are needed to make sense of the world and the people in it. This means that we trust each other with our narratives because we reveal the truths about ourselves in this way.

And so back to the story of Monkey. The four travellers had to go together. Each one on its own would not have reached the place where the scriptures were. They were on their way to find the truth that would enlighten them at home, and in the process they were enlightened. Monkey's energy was necessary; Tripitaka's understanding of the need for the journey was necessary; Pigsy's strength and concern with himself and his designed structure were necessary; and Sandy's intuition and ability to see the emergent structures were necessary. Their journey led them through a landscape that was unfamiliar, but being together they helped each other to deal with their problems of disorientation. Sandy, who had to kill to survive on earth, was 'found' by Tripitaka, the soul, and therefore did not need to kill any longer and could develop his intuition. All of them learned that life is about coping with what is given without looking for it. Life is more often living with ambiguity than certainty, searching for truth rather than 'having' truth.

Our continuing stories are never finished. The ethical responsibility lies in keeping the story going by our being involved in its creation and constantly building the metastory, envisaging the common story.

None of this is any different from other approaches to ethics, except that this one starts from the lived experience and is specifically built on and uses relationships to enhance understanding and action.

REFERENCES

Antrobus S 2000 Commissioning healthcare services: nurses as strategists, operating between policy and practice. In: Gough P, Walsh N (eds) Nursing and nurses: influencing policy, Radcliffe, Abingdon, p. 33–48

Buber M 1937 I and Thou. (Smith R G trans 1958 2nd edn, 1996 impression). T and T Clark, Edinburgh

Capra F 1998 Creativity in communities. Resurgence (186): 46–47

Donne J 1624 Devotions upon emergent occasions. Meditation XVII. In: Partington A (ed) 1993 The Oxford dictionary of quotations, rev 4th edn. QPD by arrangement with Oxford University Press, Oxford, p. 253

Doutrich D, Wros P, Izumi S 2001 Relief of suffering and regard for personhood: nurses' ethical concerns in Japan and the USA. Nursing Ethics 8 (5): 448–458

Ellis M H 1997 Unholy alliance; religion and atrocity in our time. SCM Press, London

Gadow S 1995 Narrative and exploration: toward a poetics of knowledge in nursing. Nursing Inquiry 2: 211-214

Gadow S 1996 Ethical narratives in practice. Nursing Science Quarterly 9 (1): 8–9

Gadow S 1999 Relational narrative: the postmodern turn in nursing ethics. Scholarly Inquiry for Nursing Practice 13 (1): 57–70

Glen S 1999 Health care education for dialogue and dialogic relationships. Nursing Ethics 6 (1): 3–11

Hardey M 2002 'The story of my illness': personal accounts of illness on the internet. Health 6 (1): 31–46

Haugen Bunch E 2001 Hidden and emerging drama in a Norwegian critical care unit: ethical dilemma in the context of ambiguity. Nursing Ethics 8 (1): 57–68

Maltby B, Pattison S 1999 Living values in the NHS; stories from the NHS's 50th year. King's Fund, London

Metz W 1988 From memory to writing. In: The world's religions; a Lion Handbook. Lion, Tring, p. 234

Roach MS 2002 Caring, the human mode of being: a blueprint for the health professions, 2dn edn. Canadian Healthcare Association Press, Ottawa

Sjöstedt E, Dahlstrand A, Severinsson E, Lützén K 2001 The first nurse–patient encounter in a psychiatric setting: discovering a moral commitment in nursing. Nursing Ethics 8 (4): 313–327

Thomasset A 1996 Narrativity and hermeneutics in professional ethics. Ethical Perspectives 3 (4): 168–174

Tschudin V 1995 Counselling skills for nurses, 4th edn. Baillière Tindall, London

van Hooft S 1995 Caring; an essay in the philosophy of ethics. University Press of Colorado, Niwot, CO

Veatch R M 1979 Case studies in medical ethics. Harvard University Press, Cambridge, MA

Mattering

Helen Oppenheimer

All the chapters in this book bear the authors' stamp, this one in particular. Helen Oppenheimer writes from the perspective of a Christian theologian and philosopher. She also writes about tidying the house, bears that pounce on the pavement, and cucumbers, to make her point that people matter because they mind about these things. This is a chapter about a basic philosophy of life but, in establishing this, much more comes into view. Nurses and health care professionals reading it may wonder occasionally how a particular point relates to them, only to find that the next sentence gives them the answer. Helen has a wonderful way of being immediate and relevant, even when she is writing about the most disputed topics of life in general and values of living and working together in particular.

INTRODUCTION

Ethics moves to and fro between theory and practice. One can start with a theory about what values are and go on to apply it, or start with practical activity and consider the significance of what one is doing. I am starting here from the theoretical end. I would like to commend the concept of 'mattering' as a good basis for human dealings with one another, and have a look at some problems arising from it. I believe that the practical ethics of human relations, including the ethics of nurse and patient, can be illuminated and invigorated by thinking about how people *matter*.

It is fair to state that my 'terms of reference' are Christian belief. There could be values without God, but not God without values. I would also claim, by no means paradoxically, that my approach is essentially humanist: taking 'humanism' literally, to mean committing oneself to the value of human beings, which is far from entailing the rejection of God (Oppenheimer 2001).

First, I must show what it means to treat 'mattering' as a basic concept. Secondly, I will gather up, from various places where I have tried to explain them before (Oppenheimer 1975, 1983), three fundamental affirmations: people matter; mattering matters; and mattering is more given than chosen. Thirdly, I would like to have a look at a teasing question about how to fit our values into one system; that is, about how the things that we believe matter are related (Oppenheimer 2001). I hope that this analysis may be of some interest, and even some use, to practitioners whose vocation it is to apply ethical principles to human life.

MATTERING AS A BASIC CONCEPT

I may be told, 'First define your terms'. How can I talk about 'mattering' without specifying exactly what it means? The request for a definition is not so reasonable as it sounds. Warning bells ring at the prospect of defining mattering, because mattering is not 'value-free'. 'This matters' is not a plain statement about facts: it means more than 'people get worked up about this'. There is some sort of 'ought' wrapped up in mattering and, when definitions of value words are wanted, there is a philosophical howler lying in wait.

David Hume (1739) complained about the tendency of philosophers to start with straightforward talk about facts, *is* and *is not*, and then slip imperceptibly to values, *ought* and *ought not*. His warning has been heeded. The attempt to treat values as if they were simply a kind of fact has been recognised as a logical mistake. 'This is good' is not the same kind of statement as 'this is red'. 'This is desirable' has a meaning over and above 'this is desired'.

G E Moore (1929) called the mistake 'naturalism', which means, roughly speaking, trying to make ethics into a branch of natural science. For instance, defining 'good' as what in fact makes people happy leaves the question of what ought to make them happy out of the analysis, missing the very value that the definition is trying to catch. Moore put a generation of philosophers in terror of breaking the commandment 'Thou shalt not get an "ought" from an "is"' and thereby committing what he named the 'naturalistic fallacy'.

This taboo on mixing fact and value has sometimes turned out to be more trouble than it is worth; but out of Moore's *ban* on defining a value word we can rescue a *permission* not to feel obliged to define a value word but to leave it undefined. If something is forbidden it must at least be in order not to attempt it. To refrain from providing a definition is constructive, not lazy, if the reason is that we have to start somewhere. It is philosophically respectable to lay down a foundation and build on that, rather than digging deeper and deeper into the meanings of words but never reaching bedrock.

Let me put forward 'mattering' as a basis, at the foundation, indeed, of any talk about values. If nothing mattered, there could be no good or bad, right or wrong. Here is a useful place to begin thinking about ethics. From this starting point one may set off in a direction of which Moore would hardly have approved. Whereas Moore insisted on a chasm between fact and value (is and ought), 'mattering' is a bridge-building word by which the gap can be crossed (Emmet 1966).

That something matters to someone is certainly a fact, but a fact that carries value. 'This medication has been prescribed for this patient' is a neutral factual statement, involving no value judgements. 'This medication has likely side effects' is no less plainly factual; but, for the patient, side effects matter. Side effects are not 'value-free'; they are expected to be harmful, that is, bad for us. As soon as the question is asked, 'Does this matter?', what *is* stops being neutral and overlaps with what *ought to be*.

Keeping 'ought' out of 'is' is more difficult than one may suppose. We have been taught that, first, you state the facts, being careful to leave out values: 'John married Mary'; 'They had six children'; 'They celebrated their golden wedding last year.' Then you add the value: 'Their faithful love was a good thing'; but surely the value is already included in the data? 'Celebrated' is hardly 'value-free'. What about 'John fell in love with Mary; she returned his love and they were happy'? There is no need to add, 'Good!' The value seems to be built into the given facts, inseparable like John and Mary themselves.

I am glad to align myself with those philosophers who used to be called the 'new naturalists', who linked questions about goodness and rightness with what matters to people. They risked committing the dreaded naturalistic fallacy in order to make it plain that values are not a separate world but grounded in facts. Philippa Foot (1958) for instance declared, 'I do not know what could be meant by saying that it was someone's duty to do something unless there was an attempt to show why it mattered if this sort of thing was not done' (p. 501).

If one has some idea of what human beings are, one thereby has some idea what will be good or bad for them, and therefore what their morality must be like. Not just anything can be counted as good. To be cut to the heart, literally or metaphorically, must be harmful. From people's bodily and spiritual needs there spring both limitations and possibilities for how they can flourish and therefore of what is good for them. There are restrictions upon how much it is possible for people's values to diverge. The 'new naturalists' recommended the useful notion of a 'conceptual requirement' that makes sense of value judgements by giving shape to what can and what cannot be good for beings such as ourselves, who live in one world and communicate with one another (Hampshire 1957, Hart 1961, Oppenheimer 1975).

In different historical, geographical or social conditions, different values will truly matter. Hunter-gatherer societies will have moral obligations unknown in leafy suburbs, but the structure of morality must depend upon what in fact allows people to flourish. Mattering is not arbitrary, although it can be extremely diverse.

People may value all sorts of things for all sorts of reasons, and fail to understand one another's choices; but one cannot *merely* value something apart from any kind of background (Anscombe 1957). To say 'I just choose this', and stop there, invites the question: 'What for?' Some people have sick cravings and some find themselves in exceptional situations; but it is nonsense to say, 'I choose this just because it's nasty', or 'I want this just because it's unkind', or 'This is wrong but we are never to know why.' Some story needs to be told to explain the circumstances, a story about why this matters. If I would do wrong by treading on the lines of the pavement, that is because I believe that there are in fact bears who are waiting to pounce (Milne 1924).

THREE FUNDAMENTAL PRINCIPLES

People matter

If 'mattering' is to be left undefined as a basic concept bridging the gap between fact and value, its meaning can still be shown by giving instances. Each of us has an example, or rather, *is* an example, of what mattering means (Oppenheimer 1983). I can recognise mattering in my own case and then apply it to others. I can truly say, 'I matter': here is this elementary specimen of mattering. I start by knowing one example of what I need to understand.

I like to go back to David Jenkins' Bampton Lectures, given in 1966 before he was famous as Bishop of Durham: 'I assume', he said, 'that our concern is with persons. If it is not, then I assert that our concern *ought* to be with persons'. What this assertion means is that 'every human being is under a compulsion, *both factual and moral*, to be concerned with persons.' He went on: 'You must consider in what ways it matters to you to be you, keeping your investigation in the first person' (Jenkins 1967, p. 2–3).

Derek Parfit (1984) moved from fact to value in a not dissimilar way. What matters about people does not have to be some 'deep further fact' but 'the various relations between ourselves and others, whom and what we love, our ambitions, achievements, commitments, emotions, memories…' (p. 284).

Far from it being selfish to take the way I matter to myself as given and use it as a model of mattering, this is even a Christian principle: 'Love your neighbour *as* yourself'. An earlier Bishop of Durham, Joseph Butler, declared that goodness needs more self-love not less, as well as, not instead of, more love for one another (Gladstone 1896). The value of other people does not conflict with one's own value, but presupposes it. What is sauce for the goose is sauce for the gander: that is, we are all alike in being uniquely valuable. We can interpret each other's mattering by the mattering every one of us experiences. What *love* means is entering into one another's mattering.

To understand that people who matter includes every one of us, not excepting oneself, does not do away with the practical moral problem of selfishness. The sample sum is not hard to work out: 'Someone else's mattering = my mattering'; but people fail to apply the equation, often from lack of thought and sometimes from wickedness. To be selfish is to set up a barrier, or refuse to take it down, between one's own mattering and the mattering of others. The simple step from one's own value to one another's value is blocked or anyway made more difficult than it should be. Saint Augustine had a vivid description of this state of affairs: being curved in upon oneself. One way of expressing the doctrine of 'original sin' is to say that we are born curved in upon ourselves, like home-grown cucumbers. Christian faith affirms that people can be unbent.

The principle that people matter is an improvement upon the principle, much commended by moralists, of respect for persons. 'Mattering' is warmer and more humane than 'respect' (Oppenheimer 1991). Another, grander, translation of 'mattering' is the 'sacredness' of persons. Without belittling the conviction that people are indeed sacred, it is still worth suggesting that 'mattering', as well as being more everyday and informal, is also less legalistic and potentially more comprehensive than either 'respect' or 'sacredness'.

All these ways of speaking can also be ways of talking about the soul. Souls do not have to be separate entities mysteriously attached to bodies; they are people considered as spiritual. Souls are people, looked at in the light of what matters about them. It may sound whimsical but could be enlightening to define a soul as a 'pattern of lovability' (Oppenheimer 1983, 1991).

Much of what religious people try to say about 'immortal souls' is better said in terms of people who are candidates for eternal life because they matter. It is not a necessary part of the Christian tradition that souls are immortal in the sense of being indestructible. If somebody finally refused to make the step from self-love to the love of others, the pattern of the person might be corrupted to the point of decay.

No doubt it is easier to make the move from one's own mattering to other people's if one believes in a God whose children are all precious. Believers are tempted at this point to try an argument against unbelief: we know that unlovable, unloved people really matter, but how could they, unless God loved them? Unbelievers have every right to repudiate this assumption that logically they ought to be selfish, rejecting one another as well as rejecting God. Believers are the heartless ones if they disown other people's human fellow-feeling and try to monopolize mattering.

The principle that 'people matter' leads on to all manner of arguments, practical and theoretical, about who counts as a person and about what moral conclusions follow concerning how persons are to be treated. Is it part of the meaning of 'person' that a person is a rational being? Is a fetus, or someone in a coma or who is demented, or even a pet animal, a person? Where are we to draw the line? The mattering of persons seems to have a good deal to do with being given a name to which one may respond (Oppenheimer 2001). People give animals individual names, not just 'cow' and 'dog', but 'Daisy' and 'Fido'. Identifying people in institutions by numbers is notoriously inhuman.

Questions like these about what persons are make one wonder whether there is any clear line of division between 'person' and 'not person', or whether the concept of a person could have fuzzy edges. Is being a person a matter of degree? Does one become a person suddenly or gradually? Are we endowed with personhood by God, by our parents, or perhaps by one another? Human beings seem to have a kind of responsibility to co-operate in creating one another, but how far does this responsibility extend? These are by no means academic questions (Oppenheimer 1992). Practical problems, such as allowing or forbidding abortion or euthanasia, often turn upon our understanding of what a person is.

Even if people were the only persons, it is not true that people are the only matterers. 'People matter' could be a dangerous slogan, which might seem to give human beings an unjustified supremacy. Christians have often been tempted to set up 'man's dominion' in the unfortunate sense in which human beings have assumed the right to ride roughshod over the rest of creation.

What people are is the *paradigm case* of mattering (Oppenheimer 2001). It is here that we most easily find out what mattering means, but all sorts of other beings that are not people matter too in different ways. How much wild animals matter, how much the natural world matters, are problems that have lately taken on a fresh urgency. How much works of art matter is an ancient hard question. How to relate different kinds of mattering is the teasing problem I mean to glance at before stopping.

Mattering matters

This seems an even more convincing principle than 'people matter'. It is almost a tautology, but not quite; and even tautologies may need to be reaffirmed and emphasised. Morality can hardly be understood unless the warmth and importance of 'really mattering' is found in it.

In the first half of the twentieth century the way ethics was being studied seemed to have lost the essential urgency of moral concerns. The fashionable separation of fact and value produced some analytical clarity, but at the high price of an arid detachment and a creeping moralism. There was a great deal about duty and not much about what makes life worth living. Mary Warnock, writing in 1960, pointed out the boringness of theories of ethics whose characteristic examples were the duty to return borrowed books or anyway to set oneself to return them (Prichard 1949). If that was the essence of morality, one soon began to say, 'Well, after all, what does it matter?'

Moral philosophers had got into a bad habit of abstract theorising, which paid little attention to what moral decisions are really like. Ethical discussion tended to concentrate on questions about what people could be blamed for doing or not doing. Right disappeared into rights. If one could ever go beyond duty, what one found was not human generosity but legal 'supererogation', exceeding obligation. What was not compulsory was merely optional, not compelling. It seemed naive to mention love.

In the last 50 years the idea of mattering has had a happy revival. Its enlivenment is partly due to the work of an increasing number of women philosophers, who, with no loss of intellectual rigour, put life into ethics by writing about things that really matter, using lively examples, putting their hearts into their thinking. When Mary Warnock (1960) predicted encouragingly that the most boring days were over, she found it 'agreeable to reflect that there is a great deal of moral philosophy still to be written' (p. vi). At the beginning of the twenty-first century it can be seen that she was right. One symptom of the improvement is the burgeoning of medical ethics, a subject at one time practically reduced to medical etiquette, but now lively and esteemed.

A sad qualification may be needed, that the swings and roundabouts of human fallibility have brought blame back in a practical rather than a theoretical form. The question to ask when something has gone wrong is, 'Whose fault?' and that means, 'Who is to pay?' The so-called 'culture of blame' can turn patients into litigants, letting caution seem to matter as much as care.

To say that mattering matters is a promising way of bridging the gap between fact and value. Another bridge-building word is *minding*. People matter because they mind. Both words start with facts but can be enriched by understanding that values are built into the facts.

'Mind', too, has a history of being over-theorised. Instead of exploring the way 'mind' is related to value as well as to fact, philosophers allowed themselves to be diverted into discussing something called 'the mind'. They would begin by analysing the mind in a morally neutral way, leaving out values, and then they had to ask themselves why this philosophical mind did not seem to matter enough to be worth discussing. 'The mind' became an example of the sort of empty metaphysics that has fallen out of favour since Hume, with good reason. Gilbert Ryle (1949) provided a happy image of that concept of mind as 'the ghost in the machine'.

When Odysseus visited the underworld, he had to give the ghosts blood to drink for them to become physical enough to speak to him (Homer 1967 trans). How can the ghostly minds of philosophical theory be nourished? We now have a renewed understanding that minds need bodies: that ghosts inhabiting machines are hopelessly insubstantial and ghosts separated from machines still worse.

This good emphasis upon the whole person is a start. It leads to the further perception that embodied minds (that is, people) live and act as well as think: they mind in a richer sense, and therefore they matter. To progress from minding as mental activity to minding as caring, and then from caring to loving, is not to slither down a slippery slope but to develop understanding that can be practical as well as theoretical.

To be unable to mind is pathological. The most interesting chapter in John Stuart Mill's *Autobiography* (1873) describes his near-breakdown when he realised that the utilitarianism he had been brought up to live for no longer mattered to him; and how he was cured by reading the poetry of Wordsworth. Depression in which the world seems like dust and ashes, especially when there is nothing in particular to be unhappy about, is an aspect of the problem of evil, as perplexing for people who believe in a good God as is physical illness.

In *Pride and Prejudice*, Jane Austen (1813) gave Mrs Bennet and her husband an agreeable interchange: 'If it was not for the entail, I should not mind it.' 'What should you not mind?' 'I should not mind anything at all.' 'Let us be thankful that you are preserved from a state of such insensibility' (p. 109).

'Insensibility' is absence of sensation, which, taken to its limit, is unconsciousness. It is also absence of empathy, which, taken to its limit, is cruelty. Are we to be glad that Mrs Bennet is not fainting or not heartless? If her not minding 'anything at all' means 'she is unfeeling', it is a moral indictment. To say that somebody is unfeeling both states a fact and makes a substantive moral judgement, bridging the gap, once again, between fact and value. It matters whether or not people mind. Their minding is a fact but not a neutral fact; they not only do mind, they *ought* to mind.

Refusal to mind is traditionally the deadly sin of *accidie* (indifference, torpor) (Oppenheimer 2001); it might indeed be the mysteriously unforgivable blasphemy against the Holy Spirit. Inasmuch as somebody does not mind, forgiveness is simply out of reach. It is harder to love unresponsive people than badly behaved people, and this fact has something to do with the meaning of being a person. Wilful unresponsiveness would surely be the only recognisably Christian ground for damnation. What is shocking in Albert Camus' novel *L'étranger* (1944) is not even that he has killed his mother, which here seems more pointless and incomprehensible than wicked, but that the only conclusion is his cry, 'Nothing matters'. At least it matters that some things do matter.

Richard Hare has an entertaining discussion, in *Applications of Moral Philosophy*, of 'Nothing matters', or rather, of how this dictum affected a young Swiss guest of his (Hare 1972, Oppenheimer 1983). The young man read *L'étranger* and had a sort of conversion to cosmic gloom. Professor Hare, confident that philosophy is practically useful and must have something relevant to contribute, happily persuaded the young man that he had misunderstood the logic of mattering.

Mattering, he explained, is not a mysterious process that ought to go on in the world but unfortunately does not. What does go on all the time is valuing; and to say 'this matters' means, 'I value this.' If nothing had mattered to Camus he could not have produced a work of art as good as this novel. Perhaps nothing mattered to Camus' hero, although at least he minded enough to make a point of proclaiming his discovery. So Professor Hare's young guest was easily convinced that plenty of things mattered, not because they were up to something that nobody could catch them doing, but because he valued them.

It is a pleasing piece of analysis to point out that 'My wife matters to me' is logically different from 'My wife chatters to me'. Professor Hare's explanation of the difference is that mattering 'isn't intended to *describe* something that things do, but to express our concern about what they do' (Hare 1972, p. 37–38). 'This is red' is a description; whereas 'This is good' is what Hare calls a 'prescription'. He makes *commending* a keyword, and analyses 'This is good' as 'I choose this: do so too!' (Hare 1952). This fits with the *Oxford English Dictionary's* (1961) definition of 'good': 'the most general adjective of commendation'. So far, so good: but what has happened to the idea that some things 'really matter', whether anybody is concerned to commend them or not? The question is whether Hare allows mattering to matter enough?

Mattering is more given than chosen

Professor Hare is a good representative of the kind of theory of ethics that is called 'non-objective', just because he is so evidently not an irresponsible relativist. His specific moral views should be congenial and indeed enlightening to anyone who claims to be liberal-minded. I hesitate to say that his analysis is wrong, but I do think that his emphasis on commending values as something we can choose to do is misleading and even dangerous. Values are too important to be allowed to look as if they were 'up for grabs'.

With a good deal of care, the objectivity, the 'givenness' of values may still be a good way of insisting that values matter in reality, whatever moral choices people make. Mattering is more like 'My family has a claim upon me', or 'My wife brings out the best in me', than 'I choose faithfulness.'

Hare's analysis of mattering in terms of choice goes with the way in which he distinguishes values from facts. He emphasises that it is facts that are given, whereas we have a good deal of freedom 'to form our own moral opinions' (Hare 1963, p. 2). I have dared to suggest elsewhere that this way of making the distinction should even be reversed (Oppenheimer 1983). People's active lives consist of controlling, or trying to control, facts; but values are given to them. If they decide to tidy the house or vote for such-and-such a candidate, they can get rid of the clutter or influence the result of the election. They can affect what happens, but not what ought to happen. Someone who says, 'Wasn't it amusing, he was eaten by a crocodile', can choose to make a joke, but nobody's choice can make it laughable. Could mattering not be like: 'My family has a claim upon me', or 'My wife brings out the best in me', although I cannot see anything going on?

Emphasis on choosing values is all very well if we are talking about life-styles. Perhaps it matters to me that all things shall be done decently and in order, whereas unstuffy informality matters to you and neither of us is wrong. We are allowed to decide which way of living to adopt. I have to make up my own mind whether security matters more than adventure. It is for me to choose whether my independence is worth more than my comfort, or, more toughly, whether it is worth enduring pain rather than taking mind-dulling medicine, or risk shortening my life for the sake of pursuing my dangerous goals.

A live debate today is whether questions about sexual morality ought to be treated as questions of life-style. Is living together unmarried more like starting a new job, moving house, gambling, or driving dangerously? Is divorce enterprising or treacherous, when there are no children involved? Is the diversity of people's moral lives a matter of disobedience or of creativity? How far should we criticise and how far should we honour one another's decisions?

What Hitler did to Jews has nothing whatever to do with life-style. Professor Hare is undoubtedly as sure as anyone that the Holocaust mattered dreadfully. His contention is that 'the objectivity of values' is not a useful way of putting this. Has he not, after all, blunted the edge of morality by his insistence that mattering is not a kind of activity, something things do? We cannot catch a Jewish family, or a lost child, or a cancer patient, doing something called mattering; but if we have philosophical difficulties about affirming that these matter in their own right, absolutely, quite apart from the concern anyone expresses, have we understood how much they matter?

Real mattering does not need a metaphysical world of values over and above the world of facts. It needs values built into the everyday world, values which, in some sense, are there to be found. The ethical theory that we find values by something like looking has been labelled 'intuitionism'. It may be more convincing to say that we find values by *attending*.

When I have said, 'It looks like that to me', whether about a fact or a value, it is time to ask, 'Am I seeing clearly?' Some of us have better eyesight than others, and anybody's vision, literal or moral, can be distorted in various comprehensible ways. Rose-coloured spectacles can be worn on the nose or in the imagination.

Different moral viewpoints can be compared with well-known puzzles about the experience of our senses. The straight stick looks bent in water; the round penny looked at sideways appears elliptical; the train moves away and we can see it getting smaller… These are not illusions, still less hallucinations. Far from casting doubt on the objective reality of the visual world, these are examples of how we can discover more about what things are really like by approaching them from different angles.

There is room for a good deal of variety in people's angles on the moral world. The theory called relativism is an exaggeration of the fact that much of what one sees is indeed relative to where one is. To some extent one can choose what one will see; but one does this choosing by taking up a particular stance, not by making up one's mind. People who live in the country can understand farmers better than trade unionists. Scholars can see why their own subjects matter. Teachers may judge that schools are more important than hospitals, but if they fall ill they may change their minds. One can put on blinkers, or sometimes take them off, or one can move round a bit, scrutinize closely, or stand back, but none of this means that one is free to make up one's own mind about what one will see from a particular position.

People often identify diverse values; but instead of supposing that values are therefore 'only relative', we can allow for different perspectives from which people look at the same reality. It should be possible to develop a kind of pluralism that is not relativism: a system of different values that acknowledges the validity of many points of view and recognises multifarious but objective principles.

Such a pluralism would not have to say, 'Anything goes: whatever you think is right for you *is* right for you.' It is entirely in order to criticise forms of life as just or unjust, encouraging or discouraging, cramping or sustaining, for the people who live by them. Not all points of view allow people to see clearly what is really there. Some differences of moral vision distort people's understanding, just as short-sightedness and astigmatism distort people's perception.

An objective pluralism, looking from different viewpoints at the same reality, has plenty of difficult practical problems to solve and is far from reducing moral decisions to sums with plain answers. If people are not choosing values but trying to discern them, they may find it all the more difficult to lead integrated lives. All sorts of things matter for different reasons and different kinds of reasons. Some of the most recalcitrant problems are practical questions about priorities. Of course it is hard to make up one's mind what matters most, whether one is choosing on a lofty level between the active and the contemplative life, or simply trying to decide whether to leave the washing up and play with the children. Should the patient with a wife and family, or the one who has been waiting longest, or the one who is in pain, have priority for the too-costly treatment?

There are huge questions about whether it is reasonable to have arguments about values, whether people can be right or wrong about ethical questions, or whether moral disagreements are capable of rational resolution. 'With respect', as the lawyers say, I would answer these questions with 'yes'. It would be defeatist to give up trying to give reasoned answers to questions about values. Is she an angel or a prig? Is it really a kindness to keep him happy by telling him lies? Is my vaunted integrity masking hard-heartedness? Is 'everybody does it' merely an evasion? Does his miserable upbringing mean that he should not be punished? The answers have more to do with truth than with free choice.

Because practical decisions can be right or wrong, it does not follow that all conflicts of duty are fully resolvable. I am not to say, 'I have done the sum correctly and now I can forget that problem.' Some of the values that are overridden by other values remain real and important. People's right decisions can still be tragic. Even when one would make the same decision again, it would be shallow to write off regret or even remorse as irrational (Kerr 1995).

Christians must believe that there is a 'God's eye view' (Oppenheimer 2001, p. 12), but they must not presume upon this belief. On the one hand they dare not suppose that they have a special hot-line to the truth; and on the other hand that they have no right to expect that what God sees is simple. The complexities and ambiguities of the world are as real for believers as they are for unbelievers. More happily, so are the multitudinous possibilities of bringing better out of worse and satisfying resolutions out of recalcitrant raw material, and, indeed, of bringing still richer good out of small beginnings. It would be strange if believers in a Creator had to be squeezed into a less creative morality than their sceptical friends.

INTEGRATED MATTERING

In all this I have been skirting the baffling theoretical question of how different values can at last be fitted into one system. The question of how to integrate a whole system of divers values is more theoretical than questions about, 'What shall I do now?' and may be deemed to matter less; but still the whole picture does matter. In a cool hour, when no puzzling or tragic choices immediately confront me, I can pause and think. Many things matter. Many things matter supremely. I need not rank them, but if I want to understand what to think as well as what to do, I must somehow relate them. Indeed, it should matter to students of ethics to think well as part of living well.

The many things that matter are not all compatible and a great deal depends on where I start. I have to do my best, in terms of the alternatives open to me, to achieve a satisfactory whole. However, practical wisdom will not solve the theoretical questions: How do different kinds of mattering fit into one system? How does the kind of value we call 'aesthetic' relate to moral mattering? Is it a tautology or a prejudice to affirm that morality must always matter most? If it is a tautology, it may still need explaining. If other values have some importance, even if only a lesser importance, they still need to be fitted into place.

We often need to know what to say when one claim seems to invalidate another. Suppose a good Christian writes pious trash, or we are moved by a story whose values we deplore? Are we to hang an ugly picture rather than hurt anyone's feelings, or allow people to put sentimental rhymes on their tombstones (Oppenheimer 2001)? Must we tell the truth when truth is frightening? We can say at least that what we need is inspiration rather than calculation.

The 'objectivity of ethics' is part of the problem rather than part of the answer. It is no wonder people are tempted to concede that there just is no one correct answer to questions like these and that we must decide for ourselves. This is a temptation and it can be resisted. It can still be held that, after all, right answers are to be sought, and that values are 'there' to be found rather than chosen.

Real objective mattering looks less problematic both in theory and in practice when we posit, not *something that* matters, but *someone who*. People are still the paradigm case, the main source of moral claims. People matter in the strongest sense; they matter in their own right; things matter in relation to people. This is where love comes in; the mattering of people cannot be severed from the interconnectedness of their minding.

On this basis, it may be easier to give answers, both to the practical question of what is to be done in a particular case, and also to the theoretical question of how the values fit together. The principle, 'people matter', may suggest a first step towards fitting creativity into the same system as moral goodness. Goodness, truth and beauty have to do with the fulfilment of people.

First we set up *minding* as the basis of people's mattering to themselves, to one another, and to God. The whole area we so inadequately call 'aesthetic' comes in when we go on to ask what there is for them to mind about. Instead of 'minding' we can say 'loving'. Saint Augustine (1961 trans) said 'My weight is my love.' Love cannot exist in a vacuum but has to be made actual in some sort of specific activity. As soon as we give love something to do we open the way to other valid concerns besides being good.

It is a reasonable hope that all our values may come together like this. To justify this way of integrating different kinds of mattering it would be imperative to reckon seriously with the problem of present evil, or we may find ourselves happily fiddling while Rome burns, taking short cuts to enjoyment and forgetting the troubles of other people's lives. What I am feeling for is the idea that at last the different kinds of value do not need to be rivals. Goodness is, as it were, the form, the shape, of the good life, and truth, that is reality, its condition. Then we may say that 'beauty' or 'the aesthetic' or even 'pleasure' can take its place as the substance, the stuff, of the good life.

REFERENCES

Anscombe G E M 1957 Intention Blackwell, Oxford, p.70

Austen J 1813 Pride and prejudice. (Jones V (ed) 1996) Penguin, London, p. 106–109

Saint Augustine Confessions. (Outer A (ed) 1955) SCM Press, London, p. 304

Camus A 1942 L'étranger (The stranger). (Davison R trans 1988) Routledge, London

Emmet D 1966 Rules, roles and relations. Macmillan, New York, p. 46–50

Foot P 1958 Moral arguments. Mind 67 (268): 502–513

Gladstone W E (ed) 1896 The works of Joseph Butler, vol 2: Sermons: Preface. Clarendon Press, Oxford, p. 26

Hampshire S 1957 Thought and action. Chatto and Windus, London, p. 236

Hare R 1952 The language of morals. Oxford University Press, Oxford

Hare R 1963 Freedom and reason. Oxford University Press, Oxford p. 2

Hare R 1972 Applications of moral philosophy. Macmillan: Basingstoke

Hart H L A 1961 The concept of law. Oxford University Press, Oxford, p. 176, 181–207

Homer The odyssey (Rieu E V trans 1967) Penguin, Harmondsworth, Book 11, p. 171–188

Hume D 1739 A treatise upon human nature (Selby-Bigge L A (ed) 1946) Oxford University Press, Oxford, Book 3, part 1, section 1, p. 469

Jenkins D 1967 The glory of man (Bampton Lectures 1966). SCM Press, London, p. 2–3

Kerr F 1995 Moral theology after MacIntyre. Studies in Christian Ethics 8 (1): 33–44

Mill J S 1873 Autobiography. (Laski H (ed) 1944) Oxford University Press, Oxford, p. 112–155

Milne A A 1924 When we were very young. Methuen, London

Moore G E 1929 Principia ethica. Cambridge University Press, Cambridge

Oppenheimer H 1975 Ought and is. In: Dunstan G R (ed) Duty and discernment. SCM Press, London, p. 9–22

Oppenheimer H 1983 The hope of happiness. SCM Press, London

Oppenheimer H 1988 Looking before and after. Collins Fount, London

Oppenheimer H 1991 Ourselves, our souls and bodies. Studies in Christian Ethics 4 (1): 1–21

Oppenheimer H 1992 Abortion: a sketch for a Christian view. Studies in Christian Ethics 5 (2): 46–60

Oppenheimer H 2001 Making good. SCM Press, London

Oxford English Dictionary 1961. Oxford University Press, Oxford, p. 287

Parfit D 1984 Reasons and persons. Oxford University Press, Oxford, p. 284

Prichard H A 1949 Moral obligation. Oxford University Press, Oxford, p.35

Ryle G 1949 The concept of mind. Hutchinson, London

Warnock M 1960 Ethics since 1900. Oxford University Press, Oxford

9

Whose culture? An attempt at raising a culturally sensitive ethical awareness

Sandy Haegert

Sandy Haegert believes that there are as many answers to the question of what culture is, as there are authors who have written on the subject. No doubt she is right, and she should be, if we are to follow her example. There are general ideas of what a culture is and Sandy highlights some of them with impressive clarity. There are also the personal experiences of all aspects of culture; she conveys some of these in the way she describes her own growing understanding of the subject and by urging readers directly to be on a similar journey with her. As such, the chapter itself is an experience of a culturally sensitive ethic where it is clear that living the stories and understanding their meaning is the important element.

Each particular way of knowing is supported and reinforced by human culture, and is part of the wisdom a culture transmits to its young (Lessem 1996a, p. 47).

INTRODUCTION

This chapter looks at culturally sensitive ethics from two different world-views. As a westernised white person, I am trying to look at my own culture while at the same time analysing African culture. This analysis is from my experiences of teaching and working with multiracial students and colleagues, and from books; hence my title, 'Whose culture?' If we are not ready to analyse our own culture together with its ethic then why point a finger or show up someone else's culture? We would be as guilty of ethnocentrism as any previous colonial or imperialist regime. The

context from within which I write about culturally sensitive ethics embraces work and education; the emphasis is on teaching, communication (the way we talk, and music) and management. It is about a specific world view, its values and behaviour, but it is hoped that it will also have general application.

To write of these things under the heading of culturally sensitive ethics may seem strange. However, our world of work (and with it what is transmitted) is where we spend most of our time. More than anywhere else, we meet with different cultures and confront our own ethical position most often at work. Therefore I engage with you, the reader, in dialogue about the relationship between work and ethics, and work and culture. I believe there is a point where culture and ethics merge. To engage with you in meaningful culturally sensitive ethics is equally important. I do this, notwithstanding the fact that, as Joyce Scott says, 'Beauty and meaningfulness are different things to different people' (2000, p. 11). There should be beauty and meaningfulness in culturally sensitive ethics. Scott's main thesis is that one cannot understand the value system of one's own culture until one discovers the world-view and values of another.

I use work scenarios to show what I mean and I will use other methods as I continue. Each scene, each protagonist, in the narratives portrays a particular culture; each is heavily impregnated with an ethic that weds itself to the contextual culture that can be qualified as either good or bad. These cultural stories focus on 'acts of meaning', 'communities' and ethics (Bowden 1997, Bruner 1990, Lave and Wenger 1991). The questions that I ask you to focus on as you read each narrative are: Whose culture? Whose ethic?

WHOSE CULTURE? WHOSE ETHIC?

This first scene is set in England in the mid 1970s.

We see a mother in a sluice room. A newborn baby lies on a white towel on the cold white marble; the baby, perfect in every limb, is lying motionless. No limbs flail the air, no chest movements to draw in breath—a stillbirth. The mother asks the nursing sisters accompanying her if they have a pair of scissors. The sisters look at each other. One reaches into her pocket and brings out a pair of surgical scissors. The mother puts both hands together, palms up in a gesture of thanks, and accepts them. There are no words. She turns to her baby. The sisters gather closer, watching, astounded as the mother begins to cut the infant's hair, each minuscule wisp. Then each finger- and toe-nail is gently clipped. At last, when every clump of hair and every minute nail have been cut, the mother places them on a large shawl. She stares long and hard at these tiny clippings on this huge dark surface. Then she closes her eyes. She sways back and forth. The sisters stare speechless.

Later, in telling of this lived experience they say: 'We wondered what African "voodoo" was going on. What was the reason for this odd behaviour?' These sisters had no frame of reference, no pigeon-hole into which to place this event. What they were implying was that anything African that they could not fathom out, or in their opinion 'was odd', was labelled 'voodoo'. The term 'culture' as a system of symbols reflecting socially established structures of meaning was unknown to them, as was trying to understand the culture, or way of life, of 'foreigners' or non-nationals. Only when these nurses attended a workshop on cultural diversity and learned the possible reason for the act, could they categorise this phenomenon.

The African mother had left Nigeria to study and had married. Back in her native country, a bride price had been paid. She had become pregnant. Her joy was great; fertility is ranked high in Africa. The in-laws would be pleased; the bride price was worth it. Then tragedy struck. The child died in utero. The in-laws may not believe that she had a child. What was she to do? She conceives of the idea of sending tangible evidence of a life brought forth, only to die.

Where is the culturally sensitive ethic? Focus on the nursing sisters. Focus on the cold, clinical sluice room environment in which the narrative took place. Focus on the lack of understanding and their belief systems. Notice the quick judgement, even prejudice, with what is perceived as 'odd' behaviour. In the mid-1970s any bizarre behaviour was labelled as 'odd' to explain the inexplicable. Where are the compassion, the dignified setting, the knowledge, the respect for another? These are components of ethical caring.

SOME MEANINGS

Whether we are talking specifically about ethics at work or within a particular culture we need first to ask the question: 'What is ethics?'

According to Parker Palmer (1983) ethics is to do with: the values by which we live our lives; an approach to living; and the quality of our relationships. My own meaning is that ethics form the standard of behaviour that I exercise daily towards others. I will use this last definition to formulate and discuss views on culturally sensitive ethics. I share with Ronnie Lessem (1996b) the feeling that the topic of work and education within culturally sensitive ethics must embrace 'people's vitality, their reason for being, their creativity and the spirit or soul that lies deep within each person and needs awakening' (p. 111).

Therefore, secondly, I want to raise the question: Is a work ethic different from the definition given above? I am a nurse lecturer; I teach most of the students at the college where I work on the subjects of ethos and professional practice, and I teach research to undergraduates at a university. For me, a work ethic is being able to go to work and enjoy what I am doing and for whom I am doing it because I can live by the values, and the approach to living, and the quality of the relationships I form. This means seeing and affirming the person in the students, my colleagues and my managers. It means, in setting the standard of behaviour that I exercise daily towards others, that I give and receive justice (fairness), respect and dignity. It means working for others' good (their spiritual growth), being an advocate, sharing a mutuality of caring, and showing (and receiving) ethical attentiveness, all within cultural sensitivity. In short, it means living a culturally sensitive ethic.

Where do I get these ideas? They stem from my beliefs, some of which are newly acquired through working on a PhD thesis. Ethics or spirituality are not static entities. Notice that I did not write that my ideas stem from my religious beliefs. I used the word spiritual because all of us are spiritual beings. Our spirituality is a measure of who or what we worship. As Mariana van der Walt writes: 'We define worship as the relationship I have with the person (or thing) that influences my decision-making most' (1998, p. 110). I believe, for example, that persons become (better) persons through relationships, that is, by virtue of other (good) persons. I illustrate this with another narrative.

RELATIONSHIPS ARE BOTH ETHICAL AND CULTURAL

When working as a nurse educator engaged in teaching students on the wards, the students would tell me about their experiences. One day an excellent practical nurse told me he was resigning. I asked him why. He answered: 'What is nursing? I am on this ward but I have to keep looking for procedures to fill my quota. If this is nursing I don't want it.' This second-year student was on a medical ward but the procedures he needed to practice were surgical. He had to search in other wards for patients and permission. While talking, we were approached and asked if we would see a Mr X. Nurses on this ward, including the registered nurses, all of whom were of different South African cultures, had labelled Mr X as rude and aggressive. The student and I went to the bedside and found an angry African patient in great pain, extremely anxious and highly embarrassed. Because of the removal of a rectal cancer, two drainage tubes were protruding from the patient's perineum. We were asked to attend to the surgical wound dressing.

The patient's 'rudeness' and 'aggression' was his attempt at preserving his cultural rights. In the patient's culture it is considered improper for a female (whether a nurse or not) to touch his 'private parts', no matter how necessary the intervention.

The male student nurse explained the procedure. Pain-relievers were given. With the nurse being gentle and sensitive, the patient's dignity was ensured. The patient's pain and anxiety diminished. The next day irrigations were ordered. Mr X demanded that the ward nurses find the named student to do his dressing. It was this interpretation of 'demanding' by the ward staff that had made this patient unpopular. However, on identifying the patient's socio-economic history, we discovered that in his own environment he was a chief, and so was used to influencing and controlling others.

When the student had finished, the patient asked that he should come daily. The patient was grateful because the student, by showing respect and treating him with dignity, made him feel, and I quote: 'Like a normal human being again'. Each person accepted the other. There was a sense of holism that included the cultural and spiritual parts. Previously, the student perceived nursing to be a set of procedures or tasks. He had not been given a vision of the true ethos of nursing towards vulnerable patients who need holistic care. Once he experienced the possibility of caring ethically and culturally, nursing took on a new meaning for him. His experience of being compassionately caring[1] became a growth experience for this student (and myself). As we left the patient the nurse said, 'Now I know what you mean by nursing'. He had learned the central essence of nursing—a

---

1 Care in and of itself has neither a positive nor a negative meaning. To give care or caring a positive ethical connotation, I use the term 'compassionate (or ethical) caring'.

holistic essence—its compassionate-caring ethical dimension within a different culture. In this experience something ethical (and cultural) was 'added' (Noddings 1984). The student nurse learned this meaning existentially and experientially. Through relating ethically, patient and nurse experienced 'more-being' as a person (Paterson and Zderad 1976). This nursing student finished his training with distinction.

Again, where is the culturally sensitive ethic? Ideally, all cultures honour respect and dignity, and call forth a set of techniques for adapting to 'strangers' and their immediate needs or vulnerabilities. Causing a patient embarrassment, being rude and aggressive, is so obviously non-ethical but it is also non-cultural, especially in the context of the African ubuntu (an ethical culture that will be explained later). Focusing on the student and his dilemma, this may not be the 'usual' type of ethical dilemma according to some books. However, his question about nursing is a question about ethics and culture. He is really asking: 'Is this how I and the patients I want to care for should be treated?' As Clifford Geertz (1975) intimates, elements of culture draw meaning from the roles they play and the context in which they are used. Therefore, through social behaviour and the meaning given to events, cultural forms find articulation. The behaviour of the staff revealed the ethos of that ward and their attitude. Each person's attitude arises out of his or her beliefs about the 'other'. Notice the lack of ethical compassion or cultural awareness, resulting in the unnecessary suffering of both patient and nurse.

If we are to be sensitive in a positive way to ethics and culture, then how we treat people is important. Are they like ants, mere physical workers doing repetitive tasks; or are they allowed to be themselves: creative, and developing intrinsic attitudes of accountability, responsibility and the capacity to show respect and dignity to others? What are our relationships like towards those of other cultures? Do they lack understanding? Are they harsh and impersonal? Are our relationships a type of ethical caring through which we seek to develop a person as a person?

Culturally sensitive ethical care emanates from a positive view about the human person. Inherent in this idea is that, in a relationship that involves someone (or a group), one party does not view the other as dominant or submissive. Such care is not easy; it requires much self-analysis (self-awareness and self-knowledge). Why this is so is because caring for a person should be on a deep level. Relationships in the context of culturally sensitive ethical caring embrace deep desires like trust, forgiveness, freedom, pain, hope, humility and probably others. If one has not explored these concepts oneself, one cannot help others.

What comes to mind here is the story of C S Lewis. As an academic he wrote a treatise on *The Problem of Pain* (1940). As one reads it there is a lack of compassion; it is 'head stuff'. Much later he met, and eventually married, Joy, and she died tragically of bone cancer. (Many readers will have seen the film or play *Shadowlands* by Brian Sibley (1994) about C S Lewis and Joy.) After Joy's death, he wrote *A Grief Observed* (Lewis 1966). This is a book still about the problem of pain, but written from the heart and from the depth of his own experience of the pain of grief. One senses the pain shouting at him. One feels the grief tearing at him. He shares pain with humanity. He knows. The knowledge is real, and one knows that he knows. The humanness of the person is not denied, or forgotten. It was Joy, his wife, the non-academic, who taught him the meaning of pain. He became more of a person through the experience.

If we forget another's humanness it means that we neither pay attention nor give consent (assent or affirmation) to the person being a person. We forget or lose the point that almost every person is a rational, self-aware, self-determining, free and spiritual being. The exceptions are those who are severely mentally disadvantaged. Instead of focusing attention upon the person, we often wrap ourselves in materialism, and blame 'things' for our failure to remember the person. Augustine Shutte maintains that this forgetfulness of the human person misses the most important aspect of human nature, namely the fact that we are knowing and acting subjects.

He says, 'It is our ability to think and choose that makes us not only persons but moral beings. A forgetfulness of this aspect makes it impossible either to relate morally to human nature or to give an adequate account of morality' (A Shutte, unpublished work, 1993). I believe this forgetfulness of the person has led to a crisis in modern ethics, an inability to relate morally, culturally or spiritually, and a failure to act ethically towards others.

These ideas about the person are not new. The conviction is that every human being must be treated humanely, take pleasure in a fundamental sense of trust, a ground of meaning and ultimate standards, and enjoy a spiritual home (Lessem and Nussbaum 1996).

Our sustained beliefs determine our values. My beliefs show themselves in my actions and the way I live, although, as Anne Davis states: '[These] do not always fit congruently in an action to create a moral good' (see Chapter 10). Ethical care expresses worth by embracing particular values. Morals are those fundamental principles that we believe in and live by. Ethics is the practical outworking of these morals and values. We must bear in mind that these beliefs, morals and ethics normally become public through our actions. However, many of our beliefs lie hidden or submerged deep in our subconsciousness, perhaps as unreflected aspects of our culture, or as taken-for-granted elements. Consciously or unconsciously, we share outwardly with others what we inwardly profess. We shape, and are shaped, according to our inward professions (Peterson 1983). Some may say that we are merely shaped by our culture. Culture does wield a tremendous influence over us but it need not be deterministic (a 'qué sera sera'—'whatever will be will be' sort of thing').

Therefore we need to ask: 'What is culture?' There are as many answers as authors on this subject.

CULTURE

James Spradley defined culture as: 'The knowledge that people use to interpret experience and generate social behavior' (1979, p. 5). However, rather than lean on any particular definition, let us explore different possibilities about the term and its meanings. Culture as knowledge has many forms. One can think of language, art, material things, symbolism, rules and regulations, and so on.

Culture in general is the social expression of morality: the degree of conformity to standards, principles and practice. With its socially established structures of meaning, it is also the total way of life of a people. Through culture, a particular organisation or group expresses implicitly or explicitly the ways in which its members conduct themselves in certain settings. It includes the ethos of its members, that is, a characteristic spirit or attitude, overtly or covertly prevalent in its community and transmitted to others who enter its domain. Thus, one can speak specifically of a work, or organisational, culture. Each place of work has its own culture because different members combine together, even if loosely and temporarily. They form a group through whom meaning is given: an experience is interpreted; roles are allocated, functions performed and goals achieved; and social behaviour is generated. There is group cohesion among the main characters. These are the 'insiders'. The culture is both material and non-material. The non-material is the language: written, verbal and non-verbal. There are customs and practices that are foreign to 'outsiders'. There are rites, myths and traditions. There are artefacts and symbols. There are bureaucracy, authority and subcultures. These are all evident aspects of a work culture, but each place of work is different from another. The dominant culture is expected to be learned if one is to become an 'insider' in the work-place.

To apply these thoughts about culture to a broader perspective I will use Steve Biko's (1971) ideas. Take Biko's argument and apply it to your own work situation. In doing this, you are auditing the situation to see if acculturation or accommodation of cultures applies. Where I write here of African culture, any other culture could be substituted.

AUTHENTIC CULTURAL ASPECTS

Steve Biko's ideas of culture are from his book *I Write What I Like* (2002). He felt in 1971, when he wrote the book, and South Africa was deep into apartheid, that it was most difficult to talk on anything to do with African culture with authority, because Africans then were not expected to have any deep understanding of their own culture or even of themselves. This in itself denies the fundamental characteristics of being a person. He wanted to write, or attempt to write, about the authentic cultural aspects of the African people as seen by Africans themselves. His argument was that, from his perception, Africans had experienced a one-sided approach to the process of 'acculturation' (ostensibly a fusion of different cultures). Readers, please apply this argument to your own work place. At work it may be that more than two cultures are ostensibly fused.

The two cultures that initially 'met and fused' were those of the Africans and Anglo-Boers. African culture was unsophisticated, simple and primarily relational. The Anglo-Boer culture was a method of conquest or persuasion. Their culture demanded adherence to a highly exclusive religion that denounced all other gods. No accommodation of culture was permitted. Tessa Bloem (1999) confirms this in her book *Krotoa*. Bloem is a librarian who found manuscripts pertaining to the seventeenth-century life and times of the van Riebecks. Krotoa, whom they acculturalised and renamed Eva, was of the indigenous (Khoi) people. The book could be called 'a case study in insensitive cultural work ethics'. This is what Biko is referring to when he stated that the religion of those times embraced a strict code of behaviour with respect to clothing, education, ritual and custom. This had led to feelings of superiority towards the indigenous culture. He believed that the early settlers had bestowed an inferior status on all cultural aspects of the indigenous peoples. The African culture survived only by adhering to acculturalisation strategies. Although it may have been battered nearly out of shape by the belligerent cultures it collided with, yet the fundamental aspects of a pure African culture still survive in what Biko termed 'the modern African culture' and especially in 'ubuntu'.

I use his framework, together with those of other authors, to explain his understanding of modern African culture.

THE PERSON AS SEEN IN AFRICAN CULTURE

Biko's desire was to share 'the great gift [that] still has to come from Africa'. This for him was 'giving the world a more human face' (Coetzee and Roux 1998, p. 30). For him, the ideal African society was seen as a person-centred society. This ideal is the whole crux of ubuntu. People matter more than things. This was the cornerstone of their society. Ideally, a person was not valued for his or her material, technological or social status. Rather, a person was enjoyed for himself or herself as a holistic, spiritual being. Biko's was a communal society based on the proverb-ethic: 'I am because we are' or its alternative rendition: 'A person becomes (more of) a person through other persons'. Thus, a person enjoyed for himself or herself was part of a community, part of joint community-orientated action, rather than an individual set on competing with others. Perhaps this is what Anne Davis has identified as the 'socially embedded self' of Japanese culture (Ch 10).

This concept of a person becoming a person in the context of ubuntu goes even deeper. One needs to see ubuntu as a philosophy of being, a lifestyle much like that of a Jew or a Muslim, in which one's faith and culture is inclusive of one's being and living. It was about fundamental things that qualified a person to be a person. A person was not defined as a person in the western technical philosophical sense of the term (i.e. by being rational, self-aware, self-knowledgeable, free and spiritual). If one were not seen to have the capacity for ubuntu, one would be regarded as a non-person. Through the ubuntu of others, young people were socialised from their youth up on how to be; they learned collective responsibility. The community motivated the person to respect and be respected, to be accountable, responsible and creative. It was a fountain from which actions and attitudes flowed, where the capacity for careful and courteous listening and participative consensus decision making was fostered. It was, and still should be, the bedrock of a specific life-style and culture, one that incorporated, shared and taught the ethos of not just a tribe, but Africanism itself, and its values, rhythms and culture. Ubuntu sought to honour relationships as primary, whether in a social, communal or corporate context. To give an example, ubuntu taught a person how to relate to others and their (work) surroundings, a critical factor being how to greet and not to greet them. Doing this properly indicated the humanness of the person. It gave the individual a consciousness of what she or he was able to give and/or receive.

Ronnie Lessem and Barbara Nussbaum's *Sawubona Africa* (1996) is a fascinating book, designed to educate people in management about management—specifically South African management—in what could be called a culturally sensitive ethical context. They discuss management from the point of view of a broad range of cultures, not specific cultures (like Xhosa, Italian, Japanese or West Indian) but an amalgam under the broad umbrella of a compass: namely, North, South, East and West. They use Howard Gardner's (1983) concept of multiple intelligences and seek to draw the best from them in terms of their nature and scope. What this does is take the ideal of each type's particular intelligence and apply it to a management style that is cultural in its application.

The greeting 'Sawubona' means: I see you are a human being not just because you were born but through achieving characteristics that qualify you to be regarded as fully human and a person of worth (Dandala 1996). In discussing how to greet people or companies, the Rev. H M Dandala uses the Zulu word, 'sawubona' (singular). Implied in the greeting is the desire to affirm the person's humanness. One is literally saying: I see that you are a human being, as opposed to an unwelcome spirit.' The person greeted would reply: 'Yes, I see you too are also a human being.'

What Lessem and Nussbaum (1996) do in their book about African culture is to share in particular with readers the concept 'ubuntu' and the proverb that derives from it: 'a person can be a person only through others'. They trace the treasure and richness of this African philosophy-culture and thereby 'celebrate and affirm African values'. Again, it is not that the values they celebrate are new; what they do is confirm and approve ethical values that most cultures would be glad to see in the work-place, given that the person enabling the growth of another is a positive 'ethically made' person. That person would make these ubuntu values explicit and show how they can be part and parcel of one's working life or ethos. They show that one does not have to have two sets of ethics—one for private use and another for the work-place—as I found was the case with many trained nurses when it came to practicing an ethic of care (Haegert 1999).

Biko perceived Africans as 'prescientific' people. He believed that they accepted the supernatural and non-rational as aproblematic. They allowed what they did not comprehend (a situation or irrational aspect) to impact upon them so that, by experiencing whatever was problematic or puzzling, they could make sense of it. Their response to a 'problem' or the incomprehensible is holistic; the whole personality of the individual is involved. There is an acceptance that nature has enigmas that are not 'solvable' by mere human powers. Ideally, less stress is laid on power and what it can attain, and more emphasis is put on the person. Westerners, in contrast, are geared to an aggressive analytical approach to problem solving, whereas the African attitude to this, like the concept of time, is that of experiencing a situation. Scott, for example, cites John Mbiti as saying, 'The linear concept of time, with a past, present and future, stretching from infinity to infinity, is foreign to African thinking. The dominant factor is a virtual absence of the future … to Africans time has to be experienced to make sense. The essence of time [and problem solving] is what is present and what is past' (Mbiti 1968, cited in Scott 2000, p. 42).

COMMUNICATION IN COMMUNITY

Communication embraces the way in which Africans talk to each other. Scott, in discussing cross-cultural aspects, tells about waiting an hour for a friend to arrive. Later, when the friend explained this lateness, he related that he had unexpectedly met his father and that it would have been out of the question not to spend time with him, even though he had made the initial appointment with her. She illustrates thereby the importance of communication among African family members. Two 'big' words were emphasised: 'relationships' and 'now' (Scott 2000, p. 41).

Time, Biko (1971) wrote, is taken to enjoy communication between people for its own sake and to show respect. Noni Jabavu (1960) explains: 'Culture [in the African sense] is the way we talk with people, dress, and eat' (p. 193). In writing these words, Jabavu interprets: 'the way we talk with' as meaning: '[B]eing allowed to speak without interruption, comment, comparisons; withholding, surprise or pain. Uttering only that which encourages the speaker to continue' (p. 193). I must add that, when one is sharing from the depth of one's pain or grief, to have someone listening with such ethical attentiveness is comforting. Jabavu (1960) continues: 'It is in talking that one explains artistically, poetically, properly, beautifully, in detail. This is kindness, feeling: humanity is there [ubuntu obabulapho] – it is something one can hear, if not understand' (p. 193). The use of 'talk' here, and in many other places in this work, conveys the idea of a sense of presence, finding a 'voice', even of 'a knowledge' of oneself. Timeliness (knowing the right time to do or say something) is of more value in African society than the keeping of time.

Returning to Biko (1971), he states that the term 'intimacy' was not reserved exclusively for particular friends but applied to a whole group of people who found themselves together through work or residence. He would go further and say that in traditional African culture there was no such thing as 'two friends' (a dyad). Age or division of labour (social grouping) naturally determined conversation. This was a time of commonly sharing intimacies among one's peers or colleagues. No one would feel unnecessary or an intruder. Any curiosity thus manifested would be welcome as it came out of a desire to share. House visiting was a feature of elderly folk's way of life. No reason for the visit had to be given; it was just part of a deep concern for each other. Age mates (or work peers) would share their secrets, joys and woes.

MUSIC AS COMMUNICATION

Communication with each other is not just in words but dramatised through the love of song and rhythm. Leopold Senghor summarised the connectedness of persons to the whole of life with the words: 'I feel the other, I dance the other, therefore I am' (Senghor 1956, p. 212). In South Africa many people misunderstand Africans' use of music, dance and/or drama.

According to Scott (2000), music can cause division because people misunderstand the cultural values that are expressed through this medium. A feature of all African emotional states is music (their song and dance) (Biko 1971). Through music, the emotional burdens and pleasures of work are shared. Through music and rhythm, games are played. They are part and parcel of the African way of communication, not an individual, but a communal, way of life, to share and feel the common experience, not in words but in music and movement. This is Africans' way of deriving sustenance from a feeling of togetherness and gives added energy to a situation. Music, drama and story-telling are their ways of expressing themselves with conviction and real feeling. They enhance feelings of group pride and solidarity.

Scott's thesis on music (2000) is an attempt to 'build a bridge' (p. 41) over the history of the church in Africa and the music problems involved. She wants others to recognise the value systems and world-views of different cultures and their different musical styles in order to build this bridge. She reiterates the fact that music is a well-tried African teaching method and that she has used it extensively in teaching health promotion.

PUTTING IT ALL TOGETHER

How do all these cultural and ethical ideas come together? How do we develop a culturally sensitive ethic in our nursing and in our work-place, whether college or practicum? How can we build bridges that bring distinct cultures together?

My vision for my work-place is of a cross-cultural bridge where we seek 'convergence of purpose'[2] (Knighton-Fitt, 2000, p. 185, and personal communication). There are numerous means for this: from the pragmatic use of music, dramatisation and language expression in the form of stories, to the abstract in the form of philosophy, symbolism and spirituality. We need an environment where another's culture is valued, individually and collectively. We need a philosophy of caring ethically for others: where no limit is put on human potentiality; where it is recognised collectively that each employee has a work ethic, a culture and a spirituality that needs to be realised and affirmed; and where, by creating an ethic related to the common purpose, meaning can be restored. We need to generate the meaning of a work ethic and a collective culture of development. My vision is of us trusting one another ethically and culturally.

A workshop was held at the nursing college where I work, for all managers, tutors, student representatives, housekeepers, gardeners, building workers and others, which aimed to enable staff capacity building. The facilitators found that a lack of trust was the priority problem of each group. My vision is of a college that can affirm this 'unity in diversity in education through the healing philosophy of ubuntu' (Goduka 1999, p. 2). The cross-cultural complexities of the work-place have to be understood through culturally sensitive ethical interaction. This includes the use of narrative. Peter Christie and Gina Mhlophe (1996) emphasise how stories 'help to infuse life into employees' understanding of the [work-place] culture' (p. 122). They write that 'storytelling is a powerful way for leaders to re-establish trust in

organisations' (p.129). They show that policy manuals are 'a no-no today', according to Tom Peters (1992, p. 128), a pragmatic management thinker and story-teller and that in their place is management as story-telling. 'There is a growing awareness amongst researchers', Christie and Mhlophe (1996) write, 'that management is as much an art as a science and as such should involve organisational storytelling, symbolism and the expression of language' (p. 128). I have been to a workshop where stories were told and where they produced insight, forgiveness and a new spirit of working together.

We need to demonstrate to each other that seeking for alternatives and consciously developing human potential, whether among students or tutors, is not life-threatening but can be life-releasing, setting us on a learning curve that gives new dimensions to living. How do we do all this? It can be done through creative innovation; for example, I gave a paper on 'African proverbs as a means of providing access to knowledge through language' at a conference on generating ideas for 'Integrating content and language'. I believe that we need to learn and/or teach, not only others' cultural proverbs but also their concepts, the richness of their language and the way in which words are used. In the classroom I found myself using the concepts 'ubuntu' and 'sawubona' in a discussion on human rights in the South African Constitution (South African Government, 1997) with second-year students, a third of whom were African; a few were white, and the rest were Cape Coloureds. The Africans fully understood my use of these words. I was explaining the need to see the human person in two scenarios from the news. The first was about a woman who, on World AIDS Day, had declared on television that she was HIV positive. Afterwards, her community stoned her to death. One of the African students said: 'They did not see her as a person but as an animal [less than human]; that is why she was stoned.' The other story was about people who have severe learning disabilities. Here it was told that, in order to bathe these persons, eight or ten at a time were lined up in a bath and washed as a group. With

---

2 The more preferable phrase instead of consensus is 'seeking convergence of purpose'.

the unfolding of the meaning of 'sawubona' and 'ubuntu', the class understood and correctly identified the human rights abuses taking place in these two narratives.

CONCLUSION

For there to be a culturally sensitive ethic, we need to promote harmony, but not necessarily unity. We should seek convergence of purpose and create therapeutic contexts in which we can discover the shared values, world-views, concerns and convictions of others. We should pursue the building of relationships, not the building of organisational structures. We need meaningful exchange. We need to listen, hearing not just what people say but what they mean, and what is behind what they say. We need their stories. In short, we need to be tolerant, to trust one another, and to remember that each one is a person in his or her own right.

Philosophy is made up of the knowledge and beliefs that form the values by which we 'live, move and have our being'. We become shaped by this knowledge. This, in turn, shapes our beliefs and values. As teachers and nurses we are mediators between our students and/or patients and their knowledge of a subject. The way we, as teachers and/or nurses, play this role conveys not only our epistemology but also our ethic to our students and patients. They will see what we believe, our culture and what our ethic is by the way we comport ourselves at the bedside, at the chair-side, (Ozar and Sokol 1994) or in the classroom. On a daily basis they will understand our controlling knowledge or ethic by their observation of our behaviour. Perhaps the concept of ubuntu falls short of any universal or personal ethical standard, but it is an ideal at which to aim. There is a proverb that states: 'It is better to aim high and miss than to aim low and hit spot on.'

Sawu̧bona, I see you!

QUESTIONS FROM THE TEXT

1. How would you define the term 'ethics' within your work sphere?
2. Is our work ethic different from the bioethic we hold or have learned about?
3. How do cultural and ethical ideas (theories) come together?
4. How do we develop a culturally sensitive ethic in our work-place?
5. Are our relationships culturally sensitive: a type of ethical caring through which we seek to develop another's potential within his or her own culture?
6. Can we greet one another (those of different cultures) with 'Sawubona': I see you, as a person?

REFERENCES

Biko S 2002 I Write What I Like: Selected Writings, Stubbs A (ed). University of Chicago Press, Chicago, IL

Bloem T 1999 Krotoa – Eva, the woman from Robben Island. Kwela Books, Cape Town

Bowden P L 1997 Caring: gender-sensitive ethics. Routledge, London

Bruner J 1990 Acts of meaning. Harvard University Press, Cambridge, MA

Christie P, Mhlophe G 1996 Management as storytelling. In: Lessem R, Nussbaum B (eds) Sawubona Africa – embracing four worlds in South African management. Zebra Press, Sandton, p. 122–135

Coetzee P H, Roux A P J (eds) 1998 Philosophy from Africa: a text book with readings. International Thompson Publishing, South Africa, p. 26-30

Dandala H M 1996 Cows never die: embracing African cosmology in the process of economic growth. In: Lessem R, Nussbaum B (eds) Sawubona Africa – embracing four worlds in South African management. Zebra Press, Sandton, p. 69–84

Gardner H 1983 Frames of mind. Fontana, London

Geertz C 1975 The interpretation of cultures. Hutchinson, New York

Goduka I N 1998 Educators as cultural awakeners and healers izangoma: indigenising the academy in South Africa. South African Journal of Higher Education 12 (2): 49–59

Goduka I N 1999 Affirming unity in diversity in education: healing with ubuntu. Juta, Kenwyn

Haegert S 1999 A critical analysis of the concept care in the practice and discourse of nursing [thesis]. University of Cape Town, Cape Town

Jabavu N 1960 Drawn in colour – African contrasts. John Murray, London

Knighton-Fitt J 2000 One evangelical's experience of the parliament of world religions. South African Baptist Journal of Theology 9: 185–188

Lave J, Wenger E 1991 Situated learning; legitimate peripheral participation. Cambridge University Press, Cambridge, MA

Lessem R 1996a South Africa's multiple intelligences. In: Lessem R, Nussbaum B (eds) Sawubona Africa – embracing four worlds in South African management. Zebra Press, Sandton, p. 47–61

Lessem R 1996b Case-study: Cashbuild reinvents itself. In: Lessem R, Nussbaum B Sawubona Africa – embracing four worlds in South African management. Zebra Press, Sandton, p. 110–116

Lessem R, Nussbaum B (eds) 1996 Sawubona Africa – embracing four worlds in South African management. Zebra Press, Sandton

Lewis C S 1940 The problem of pain. Geoffrey Bles, London

Lewis C S 1966 A grief observed. Faber, London

Mbiti J S 1968 Eschatology from African concepts of time. African Theological Journal (Makumira, Tanzania). In: Scott J 2000 Tuning into a different song – using a music bridge to cross cultural differences. Institute for Missiological and Ecumenical research, Pretoria

Noddings N 1984 Caring: a feminine approach to ethics and moral education. University of California, Berkeley, CA

Ozar D T, Sokol D J 1994 Dental ethics at the chairside: professional principles and practical applications. Mosby, St. Louis, MO

Palmer P J 1983 To know as we are known – a spirituality of education. Harper and Row, San Francisco, CA

Paterson J G, Zderad L T 1976 Humanistic nursing. John Wiley and Sons, New York

Peters T J 1992 In search of excellence. Harper and Row, New York

Peterson E H 1983 Run with horses: the quest for life at its best. Inter-varsity Press, Downers Grove, IL

Scott J 2000 Tuning into a different song – using a music bridge to cross cultural differences. Institute for Missiological and Ecumenical Research, Pretoria

Senghor L 1956 L'esprit de la Civilisation ou Les Lois de la Culture Negro-Africaine, vol VIII-X, Paris. In: Lessem R, Nussbaum B (eds) 1996 Sawubona Africa – embracing four worlds in South African management. Zebra Press, Sandton

Sibley B 1994 Shadowlands: the story of C S Lewis and Joy. Hodder, London

South African Government 1997 The South African Constitution [501D-E]. Government Printing Press, Pretoria

Spradley J P 1979 The ethnographic interview. Holt, Rinehart, and Winston, New York

van der Walt M 1998 Ministering to people from a homosexual background: a biblical framework. South African Baptist Journal of Theology 7: 103–120

10

International nursing ethics: context and concerns

Anne J. Davis

An international ethic has to consider culture, but cultures differ. Anne Davis draws on her wide international working experience to write about an increasingly puzzling area of nursing: can the same standards and principles apply everywhere? This chapter does not provide an answer to the question, but an important critique of what an international and cultural approach can do or achieve. No one can avoid cultural influences, just as all our work is international. The more we learn, the more we know, but Anne asks us to learn sensitively, with respect, mindful of the way in which we create cultures and ethical norms.

INTRODUCTION

One Sunday I attended mass in the Catholic Church of Arezzo, a lovely small city in Tuscany, northern Italy. I actually entered the church to view the famous Piero della Francesca frescoes and, when mass began, decided to stay. A few weeks earlier, while still living in a small town in central Japan, I visited the beautiful local Buddhist temple. Being neither Catholic nor Buddhist, I probably experienced these visits differently from those who share these belief systems. Both visits gave me some quiet time to think about things beyond the ubiquitous, mundane concerns of daily life. As I looked at the quiet but commanding austerity of the temple and the Gothic simplicity of the church, now embellished by religious artifacts, each so extremely different from the other, I wondered if those who usually come to worship at these sites

see the world through other cultural lenses than the ones I have and, if so, what their lenses reveal to them. As I thought about these possible differences, I began to extend my thinking beyond religion to other influences that create a person's world-view. This extension resulted in the conceptual organisation for this chapter.

Every person is born into a culture, joining an ongoing stream of sociocultural definitions and arrangements that make living together in a group possible. This stream seems stable and dynamic at the same time, stable in its core foundation but dynamic as it reacts to change. Such change can modify the core foundation, but aspects of it remain over long periods of time.

This chapter discusses international nursing ethics from the perspective that all people exist in their taken-for-granted culture and have attending world-views that seem natural and normal to them, and which may differ significantly from my own. In taking this approach, I raise questions and concerns about nursing ethics from an international perspective. First, I need to set the contextual stage for these questions and concerns.

CULTURAL PRACTICES AND MORAL AUTHORITY

Think how wondrous and richly diverse the world really is and how the global village of our present day world makes possible our knowledge of many other cultures, including those in the most remote areas of our planet. We can learn about the nomads in Mongolia, the community tribal sing-sings in Papua New Guinea, the former headhunters in Malaysian Borneo up-river from Kuching, as well as about people who live in Paris, Beijing, Bogotá, New York, Nairobi, Delhi and Moscow. This learning can be vicarious or from direct experiences, or both. We can obtain it from the mass media, reading, discussions with others, and travel. I have visited people in and read about all these places, and many more around the world and, from these remarkable experiences over the past 40 years, I realise how both similar and different humans have become, as people live in cultural groups on different continents. Within these groups, people have their culturally defined world-views that include beliefs, values, and social definitions and arrangements.

When teaching at the University of Ibadan, Nigeria, in 1971, I was told that a young child stood in the middle of her tribal village, stamped her foot, and asked, 'Just who is my mother?' Her experience of receiving care and attention from all the village women made identifying her biological mother difficult. Although such a social arrangement functions to help these women to complete their daily work, it can also raise questions about mother–child bonding as a value in some cultures, which has interested nurse practitioners and researchers. How do we view this story? How should we view it ethically? What do we understand about the complex dimensions of these cultural definitions of tribal relationships and child rearing practices in that culture?

Another example, and a more dramatic one, focuses on what the World Health Organization (WHO) calls female genital mutilation (FGM), a widespread practice in some parts of Africa, Asia and the Middle East. This practice, formerly referred to as female circumcision, is often performed with crude and unclean tools and functions to keep females sexually pure for marriage when they become older children or young adults. It can also do great physical damage to these girls; some will die as a result, while others will have health problems throughout their lives (Davis 1998). The same

questions as above can be asked: How do we view this practice? How should we view it ethically? What do we understand about the complex dimensions of culturally defined gender roles and this cultural practice?

When I taught an ethics course at a nursing college in Japan, I used this example and asked third-year undergraduates what they thought would be an ethical response. Some students said this practice should be viewed as unethical and such organisations as WHO should pressure governments to take action to end it. As they described their reasons for their ethical position, they talked about the great and lasting harm done to these female children. Other students, equally repulsed by this practice, saw it as an integral part of these cultures and, as outsiders, they considered that they had no moral authority to take a position on this practice. In fact, to do so would itself constitute an ethical problem (Davis et al 1999).

These students' ethical positions on this cultural practice reveal the heart of the ethics questions and concerns that will occur if we attempt to develop in-depth international nursing ethics. If universal human rights and universal ethics do exist then one can argue that such a harmful practice should be eliminated using these universal values. This argument immediately raises the question of whether we have these universals or not. What cultural and historical sources do we find here? Put another way, who decided the value content of these universals and where did they get these values?

The flip-side of this argument quickly emerges and we must ask: If we have regard for the integrity of a culture, should we, as members of another culture, assume moral authority in our view of and suggested actions towards this practice? This raises the next question: Do we live in a world where anything goes, where all cultural actions and arrangements within a specific culture, no matter what they are and what consequences they have, can be considered of equal moral value and equally morally acceptable?

Sometimes, when health professionals discuss such a cultural practice within an ethics context, someone will say that this practice is very complex and we need to understand it more before we rush to judgement. In this case, WHO has ample data on the health consequences of FGM. More than 84 million women now living have undergone this painful, frequently unsanitary, often harmful, maiming custom that can lead to the death of the female child having the procedure forced on her (World Health Organization 2001). We need to ask whether obtaining more understanding is in itself enough or can this serve to dismiss the possible ethical and human rights issues involved? Do we address the ethical dimensions of this practice when we limit our actions to more discussion to gain additional understanding of the health consequences already widely documented by WHO? Yes, we need all the information, knowledge and understanding that we can muster before questioning or condemning a cultural practice in our own or another culture. The question before us at this juncture becomes where we should draw the line between being tolerant and respectful of cultural differences, and of being intolerant of a specific cultural practice and taking an ethical position against this practice that many see as an unethical infringement of human rights.

TOLERANCE AND INTOLERANCE

As children, our parents teach us to respect the differences we encounter in other children. Such teaching includes respect for children of different colour and religion, children with accents or who dress differently, etc. Early in life many of us learn to value these differences and we try to respect them in our daily lives. As adults, this valuing with respect is not always so easy when we live in social environments where prejudices exist and, at times, permeate the social fabric of life. The important point remains that many of us have a general belief that respecting cultural and racial differences is a moral good, and that not to respect them constitutes a moral failure. Such a belief does not prevent us from discriminating against those who differ from ourselves and of thinking that they have less

social or personal worth as people. Beliefs, values and actions do not always fit congruently in an action to create a moral good, but when we confront a cultural practice in another culture that differs from our own, we may hesitate to question it and even more so to condemn it. To do so makes us seem intolerant of cultural differences. In the meantime, many ethically questionable and even problematic practices occur internationally, such as capital punishment, easy access to guns, FGM, etc.

Where should we draw the line between the general value of tolerance for differences and being intolerant of specific cultural behaviour and practices deemed to be unethical? Without some idea of basic values that apply to all, we could not have the concept of human rights. The United Nations has worked diligently to develop positions on human rights that apply in all cultures across all countries. One criticism of these documents can be found in the belief that western philosophical and religious ideals frame the content of these United Nations human rights documents, so that they contain biases or values that do not always fit with non-western cultures.

This fundamental problem of how to balance the general value of tolerance for cultural differences with the questioning or condemning of cultural practices differing from one's own remains a central issue in discussions of human rights and international ethics, with ramifications for health care and nursing ethics, especially in the international arena. Some years ago a popular saying was that: 'If you don't stand for something, you will fall for anything.' In other words, without some basic global values, anything goes and can be justified as morally permissible, if not actually being a moral good. Furthermore, you will surmise that, because a specific practice occurs within a culture, you have to believe that it can be ethically justified.

Such thinking becomes reinforced by the modern concept of the nation state. Governments and history place artificial boundaries around land and then declare it a specific place with a specific name that often only war can change. We have inherited the idea of the sanctity of the nation state, so while atrocities happen in one nation, other nations look on with impunity. This may change with globalisation when the boundaries of nations' self-interest lessen or become more porous.

The Cold War era, which dominated the world from the end of World War II in 1945 to the fall of the Berlin Wall in 1989, represented a time of clashing values between communism and capitalism, and can be depicted as a time of division. When taken together, the elements of the Cold War system influenced the domestic politics, commerce and foreign relations of virtually every country in the world. Thomas Friedman (2000) notes that the new international system, replacing the Cold War, called 'globalisation', depends on integration of markets, nation states and technologies to a degree never witnessed before. However, as this author continues, the world does not contain only microchips and markets, but also women and men with all their peculiar habits, traditions, longings and unpredictable aspirations. We have a world as new as the Internet web or a Lexus car and as old as a gnarled olive tree on the banks of the Jordan River in the Middle East. We now live in a world with great pressures towards international integration versus pressures to retain age-old cultural values and traditions.

It has become difficult for average people with money to invest to know about the companies they invest in, while, at the same time, more and more people in both industrialised and non-industrialised countries are investing. Who owns what company and what values, other than making money, may they have? Where does the food we eat come from and who harvests it, working under what conditions? Where do our clothes come from and who makes them, in what working conditions? What happens in the South American rain forest; who benefits and who is harmed by the actions taken? What does it take to get nation states to agree on issues surrounding global warming? How do the answers to all these questions and any possible

international policies addressing them affect the health status of the world's populations? How does the world's health status affect one nation state? An important question is: What beliefs, values and world-views become paramount in the decisions made?

This discussion on tolerance and intolerance of cultural differences within the larger recent economic and social changes may seem far removed from the topic of international nursing ethics, but this is actually not the case. Rather, in order to understand international nursing ethics, and any other international aspect of life, we need to understand the world in which we live. Even those people who are least affected by the global shifts will be drawn into these changes. All such massive socio-economic shifts, and their attendant changes, influence the way we view our world, how the various parts of the world interact with one another, and what becomes important to maintain and what becomes necessary to modify or eliminate.

An example can be found in the fact that English has become the international language of science, commerce, technology and diplomacy. In Japan, where the language structure differs greatly from English, some people have voiced concern about the impact of so much English on their own culture and the possible loss of ancient Japanese traditions and values causing modification of their culture in some fundamental ways. In addition, much discussion is under way about disclosure of medical information to patients and not just to their families, and about culturally sensitive forms of informed consent. As a society of obligation, Japan finds itself infused with notions of individual rights that mostly came from the West. Some Japanese fear that these notions will weaken or completely eradicate some traditional cultural values and traditions. How can Japan, and other cultures, maintain their cultural identity and integrity while at the same time actively participating in the world as it has become in this new era of globalisation? How does all this relate to international nursing ethics?

FOUNDATIONS OF ETHICS AND HEALTH CARE ETHICS

In order to raise questions and voice some concerns about international nursing ethics, it becomes necessary first to comment on the ethical foundations of western bioethics. This has been a dominant force in the field internationally and has greatly influenced nursing ethics. The usual secular categories of theories of ethics include virtue ethics, principle-based ethics, communitarian ethics and, more recently, caring ethics and feminist ethics. Many of these theories have been infused with ideas and values from the western philosophical perspective since the time of the early Greek thinkers. The definition of the individual as a separate person with a self constitutes another important philosophical definition central to western ethics, and therefore to western bioethics and nursing ethics. Those whom society defines as being a self or as having personhood can make certain claims on that society; they have rights. Although we have sensitivity towards non-human animals, we have historically viewed them as lacking personhood or a self. They have value, but often this amounts to an instrumental worth because we value them for what they can do for us and not simply for themselves.

In the late seventeenth century, John Locke tried to answer the question of what makes for a moral distinction between non-human entities and ourselves. He wrote in his *Essay Concerning Human Understanding* that the following elements made us human and different from non-humans: intelligence, the ability to think and reason, the capacity for reflection, self-consciousness, memory and foresight (Locke 1690). Although these elements do not lack problems, the West has used them to a very large extent in defining the person. This defines the individual self and not the relational self, although one can argue that, to be relational, a person must possess these elements. The myriad of questions that this western definition raises must be left without further discussion here. The point remains that this cultural definition, the social constructions of the self, varies considerably across cultures.

All cultures form some concept of the person but these definitions differ. For example, the western definition of self, based on liberal individualism, differs from the Confucian relational concept of the person that has greatly influenced Asia and accounts for the Japanese word for self that means the socially embedded self and not the individual self (Ci 1999, Harris 1999, Rosenberger 1992).

The western values and ideals both influenced and were influenced by the Jewish and Christian religions. These foundational influences became part of western thinking early in the development of the history of ideas. Religious ethics, developed from within a particular religious dogma, such as Catholic ethics, Buddhist ethics, Hindu ethics, and Islamic ethics etc., influenced the people living in those areas where they became dominant.

All cultures have within them ideas of right and wrong, good and bad, integrity and compassion, obligations and legitimate claims. All world-views held by cultural groups contain these ideals. How each culture defines these ideal values and the boundary of each one differs, depending on the historical influences, such as religion and secular philosophy that have acted upon them.

Health care ethics, including nursing ethics, can best be understood in depth only within this larger sociocultural and historical context. International nursing ethics can be understood only from within this frame. This larger view helps us to understand why we value what we value, and why what we value may differ from what others in another culture value. It is important that this view helps us to draw the line between being tolerant and respectful of culturally different values and having some sense of what we can legitimately question and even condemn as unethical. For the latter, we need to know as much as possible about the influences behind the cultural values and ideals.

For example, to support FGM, some say that the Islamic holy book, the Qur'an (Koran), approves of this practice. I personally cannot read the Qur'an in Arabic, but those who can, tell me that it does not support this practice. Other examples include the following. Although slavery has been a tradition in numerous places since ancient times, including the Greece of Aristotle, Socrates and Plato, the Roman Empire, and the nineteenth-century US south, tradition does not make slavery morally right. Many people would react negatively to the idea that slavery can be ethically justifiable because it is integral to a culture. Most of us would be greatly offended by a policy proposal to use non-voluntary active euthanasia to shorten the life of all persons aged over 90 years of age in a particular culture. Most of us would be morally concerned by women's utilitarian reproductive function depicted in the powerful novel, *The Handmaid's Tale*, by Margaret Atwood (1998). We refer to these reactions as moral intuition. Although we may not be able to tell another person why we react in this way, we have awareness of our strong feelings that something is wrong. In each of these examples we find the lack of respect for persons to be ethically problematic, whether we can use that concept verbally or not.

We often experience something terribly amiss in such situations and respond with moral intuition to the issues because we have absorbed our cultural ideals of right and wrong without always knowing the content of this socialisation or the extent to which it creates our own world-view. We all resemble a fish in water that has no reason to question its view of the norm. This is true of all people in all cultures; the ethical foundations of my culture, whatever they may be, are for me the norm. I am a fish in my cultural water and you are a fish in your cultural water. To the extent that your culture differs from mine, I can view you as a fish in strange water or a morally-suspect water. Perhaps, I view you as something other than fish. Historically, and even today, people sometimes simply dismiss others who differ from themselves as non-persons. In war, an enemy becomes a non-person whom it may be ethical to kill. We can see others as inferior to ourselves because of their race, class, religion, gender or culture. If and when we have these views and

an awareness of them, we need to stop and try to examine them, and understand how we arrived at our view. Such views can be found among members of the nursing profession, both within cultures and across cultures.

VARIATIONS WITHIN CULTURES

To this point, I have discussed culture as if each cultural group is homogeneous and all members of any such group think about and view the world in a similar fashion. In reality, as we all know, life is never this simple. Within cultures one can find divergent ethical positions on the same issue: people with similar thinking about an ethical issue reaching different conclusions; and people with different thinking about an ethical issue arriving at the same conclusion.

As an example of this within-culture variation, I will discuss the ongoing debate surrounding death and dying in Japan that has been under way for approximately four decades. I draw these remarks from two sources. The first, my own experience of conducting research on ethical issues surrounding death and dying in Japan for five years, gives me insights into this subject (Davis 1999, Davis and Konishi 2000, Davis and Mitoh 1999, Davis et al 2000, Konishi and Davis 1999). The work of Susan Long, an American anthropologist who conducts research in Japan, provides the second source. Japan, as a case study in this chapter, illustrates cultural differences and within-culture variations, but these concepts are not unique to any one country.

Japan, like all other cultures, has complexities and contradictions within it, created by many factors including: differences of opinion between and among people and groups, urban/rural adherence to traditional or modern values, and generational/gender perspectives that differ on important matters. Ambiguity, a normal part of daily life anywhere, results from these complexities and contradictions. In Japan, one can experience an ancient Shinto shrine alongside a late twentieth-century office building already reaching well into the future, or one woman in kimono and another in jeans and a T-shirt waiting for the same bus. This juxtaposition of ancient and modern, a symbol of a strong traditional culture alongside the latest faces of modernity, reflects the struggle to maintain the one while embracing the other. A gap exists between the ideal and the reality that, of course, is not unique to Japan, a very homogeneous culture with great pressures for maintaining conformity.

Public discussion on end-of-life issues reveals multiple values and world-views that make arriving at a social consensus on end-of-life ethics difficult, if not impossible. Some think that 'death education' will help to create a consensus, but others wonder if deeper sources of conflict remain that undermine such efforts.

Susan Long explained the diversity in the Japanese perspective as follows: like most people, the Japanese do not go through life as assembly-line objects; personal ethical dilemmas pit equally central values against each other, causing any resolution to be temporary and unsatisfying.

At the social level, multiple and divergent ideas that apply to end-of-life decisions provide a range of interpretative options for people socialised to their meanings (Long 2001).

The Japanese language has no word for 'dying' but the various words that the Japanese do use when thinking about dying are symbolically powerful ways that capture the range of associations that people have with dying. These associations differ and lend themselves to ambiguity in an uncertain world. Another source of ambiguity lies in the fact that contradictions can be found among equally culturally valid ideas about interpersonal relationships. Many people support the value of respect for individual autonomy and some social movements advocate the rights of patients, usually in the context of disclosure of diagnosis and informed consent. However, placing the patient at the centre of decision making contradicts other values and messages in Japanese culture. Good care-givers, whether health professionals or family members, should provide services to deal with bodily needs and also maintain a calm emotional environment. Many care-givers take this to mean that patients should not be forced to deal with bad news or to

make difficult decisions. Good care-givers protect patients (Long 1997). Some say that, because of this interpretation, many prefer non-voluntary euthanasia to voluntary euthanasia, and mercy killing is not always distinguished from active euthanasia (Hoshino 1996, Tanida 1997).

Spiritual traditions help to create attitudes and assumptions about dying and death, providing another source of mixed messages for the Japanese. Buddhist, Shinto and Bushido, as the major spiritual traditions, do not always agree, either within their own belief system or across these traditional systems, about the right actions surrounding death, including suicide. Furthermore, some think that the Japanese attitude towards dying and death is communal and does not involve a strong fear of death (Maruyama 1999), but not everyone would agree with this ideal view and some research indicates otherwise (Long 1999). The role of ancestors and spirits remains strong in Japan and helps to shape people's attitudes about dying and death. A 1995 newspaper poll found, in response to questions about human souls continuing after death, 50% said 'yes', 38% said 'no', and 12% gave another answer or did not respond (Anonymous 1995). In 1994, another newspaper poll asked people if the souls of the deceased watch us, and 89% said yes (Anonymous 1994). The living and the dead remain connected through mutual dependency (Smith 1999).

This brief and somewhat simplistic discussion of factors in Japanese culture, often viewed as homogeneous and conformist, shows just how complex cultural and ethical interacting factors can be. The central ideas here, not unique to Japan, can be found in some form in most cultures. When thinking about international nursing ethics, such factors as ambiguity and uncertainty within a culture need our attention or we can easily fall into responding to stereotypes. These comments on cultural practice and moral authority, tolerance and intolerance, foundations of ethics and health care ethics, and variations within a culture, give us a frame within which to think about international nursing ethics.

INTERNATIONAL NURSING ETHICS

This chapter has focused at some length on the larger context in which ethics, health care ethics, and nursing ethics develop and function. The necessity to understand this larger context, and the influences found there, is of paramount importance in any serious deliberation on international nursing ethics. Shifting to international nursing ethics as the central focus, the immediate concern becomes what nursing means by the term, 'international nursing ethics'.

One meaning implies that all nurses in all cultures have identical or closely akin professional values and ethics to guide their practice in the clinical, educational and administrative arenas. The International Council of Nurses *Code of Ethics for Nurses* implies this meaning in its very existence. Like all professional codes, the Code can provide only general statements on various values that are important to nursing, but cannot deal with specifics (International Council of Nurses 2000). One mark of a profession is a code for its members. As important as professional codes are, however, they cannot inform nurses with any specificity as to the right action in a particular situation. Nurses must think through each situation, drawing from a repository of knowledge, cultural and professional values, and a sense of professional responsibility.

Another interpretation of this term, international nursing ethics, could mean that all nurses in all cultures do share the same professional values and ethics, but the content of these values and ethics differs considerably. These differences in the meaning of fundamental nursing values and ethics arise from the larger context of cultural differences discussed above. Many nurses in diverse cultures would say that nurses should be caring and therefore use caring ethics as their guide for practice, but what may this really mean?

For example, in the USA, a caring presence may mean being open and honest with patients, talking with them about their health status, including their terminal illness. In Japan, a caring presence may mean being closed to certain topics and attitudes in order to withhold information from patients (especially that concerning terminal illness), maintaining a calm environment, and not unduly burdening the patient. These possible differences between the USA and Japan show opposite meanings of caring. In Japanese, no word for 'caring' exists so when describing it, nurses must use other words, usually virtues such as kindness, empathy and gentleness. Caring, a complex ethical ideal, does not translate easily into all languages and may mean other than what it does in English, the language in which caring, as a basis for ethical thinking and actions in nursing, was theoretically developed. In addition, given cultural differences, various cultural meanings extending beyond language translation problems remain, even in those situations of similar language. These remarks can also be said of virtue ethics, principle-based ethics, communitarian ethics and feminist ethics. What content do these theories of ethics contain, as they move across cultures? It is important to ask: can and should these theories developed in the West, and presented here, be the only ways to think about international nursing ethics? Perhaps other theories at present unknown to us could provide a valuable new view of the concept.

Another meaning of international nursing ethics has a darker side that we seldom admit to or examine openly. It could mean that nursing ethics, as developed in the English speaking West and exported around the world, with all the culturally defined values and notions of the self, is simply there as the only possible or the only true definition. Should this be the standard for evaluating the ethics of nursing actions in all cultures? The unspoken idea here is that, once nurses in other cultures become as morally developed as we in our English speaking cultures have become, they too will be ethical. This may reflect a search for universal values and a universal nursing ethics containing the same meanings regardless of cultural differences (Davis 2001). This would mean that nursing wants the content of international nursing ethics to be universal and western, while at the same time it admits to cultural differences. In this we have created a nursing world of cultural pluralism and western ethics as universals. Is such a creation possible? This thinking may also reflect other assumptions that are at best naive and, at worse, uninformed and arrogant.

INTERNATIONAL NURSING ETHICS: A SUMMARY OF CONTEXT AND CONCERNS

This chapter has attempted to address some complex questions of context and concerns in international nursing. In examining the context, several concerns arose. They are as follows:

1. The first and most fundamental concern is the question: 'What exactly do we mean by the term 'international nursing ethics'? The need for clarity has become apparent. If nursing continues to use this term, then more thinking through of the possible assumptions, values and differences within world nursing needs much more serious discussion, dialogue and debate.
2. A second concern has to do with moral authority and who has it on what grounds. In any given culture, the playing field is rarely even for all the players. Older people and/or males often hold social positions of authority that also include moral authority. They become the voice of the family, community and nation. The concern here is how they attain, maintain and use such moral authority, and the consequences of this sociocultural arrangement.
3. Another concern focuses on being tolerant and respectful of cultural differences, while at the same time condemning some action in another culture as ethically wrong and acting to eradicate it. The ethical tension is how to balance tolerance of cultural differences with specific unethical cultural practices as defined by someone outside the culture under scrutiny.
4. The fourth concern has to do with nursing ethics theories, especially those developed in the West and then imported abroad. The concern arises whether, in this era of globalisation, more influence from the West will dominate. The ethical question is: 'Should it?'

I hope that this wider view of international nursing ethics and the selected concerns outlined here will assist the nursing profession in many cultures, as well as nursing's international organisations, to grapple with these and other questions about international nursing ethics in the spirit of tolerance and respect for the purpose of further developing the nursing profession.

QUESTIONS FOR REFLECTION

1. How do we respect another culture while at the same time saying that some of its practices are unethical?
2. Was Dante correct when he said that the hottest place in hell is for those who stand by and do nothing when something unethical occurs?
3. Are there universal values, ethical standards of behaviour, and definitions of the self?
4. Are there any possible problems with human rights as used by international organisations?
5. Can different countries maintain the integrity of their values and traditions in a world of globalisation?
6. In what ways could globalisation affect the ethics of health care and nursing?
7. What is the foundational knowledge of nursing ethics, and can it be international?
8. What do you mean by the term 'international nursing ethics'?

REFERENCES

Anonymous 1994 Poll on Japanese attitudes about the dead watching [newspaper article]. Yomiuri Shimbun Jun 23, p. 1 (in Japanese)

Anonymous 1995 Poll on Japanese attitudes about souls after death [newspaper article]. Ashai Shimbun Sep 12, p. 1 (in Japanese)

Atwood M 1998 The handmaid's tale. Anchor Books, New York

Ci J 1999 The Confucian relational concept of the person and its modern predicament. Kennedy Institute of Ethics Journal 9 (4): 324-346

Davis A J 1998 Female genital mutilation: some ethical questions. Medicine and Law 17 (1): 6–10

Davis A J 1999 Global influence of American nursing: some ethical issues. Nursing Ethics 6 (2): 118–125

Davis A J 2001 Ethics in international nursing: issues and questions. In: Chaska N (ed) The nursing profession: tomorrow and beyond. SAGE, Thousand Oaks, CA, p. 65–73

Davis A J, Konishi E 2000 End of life ethical issues in Japan. Geriatric Nursing 21 (2): 89–91

Davis A J, Konishi E, Mitoh T 2000 Rights and duties: ethics at the end of life in Japan. Eubios Journal of Asian and International Bioethics 10 (1): 11–13

Davis A J, Mitoh T 1999 Dying in the USA and Japan: selected ethical and legal issues. International Nursing Review 46 (459): 135–138

Davis A J, Ota K, Suzuki M, Maeda J 1999 Nursing students' response to a case study in ethics. Nursing and Health Sciences Journal 1 (1): 3–6

Friedman T L 2000 The Lexus and the olive tree. Anchor Books, New York

Harris J 1999 The concept of the person and the value of life. Kennedy Institute of Ethics Journal 9 (4): 293–308

Hoshino K 1996 Euthanasia in Japan: update. Cambridge Quarterly of Healthcare Ethics 5 (1): 144

International Council of Nurses 2000 Code of Ethics for Nurses. ICN, Geneva

Konishi E, Davis A J 1999 Japanese nurses' perceptions about disclosure of information at the patient's end of life. Nursing and Health Sciences 1 (3): 179–187

Lock J 1690 Essay concerning human understanding, Pringle-Paterson E S (ed) Clarendon Press, Oxford (reprinted 1964)

Long S O 1997 What is ideal caregiving? Japanese ideals and reality from an American's perspective. Hosupisu to Zaitaku Kea (Hospice Care and Home Care) 5 (1): 37–43 (in Japanese)

Long S O 1999 Family surrogacy and cancer disclosure in Japan. Journal of Palliative Care 15 (3): 331–342

Long S O 2001 Ancestors, computers, and other mixed messages: ambiguity and euthanasia in Japan. Cambridge Quarterly of Healthcare Ethics 10 (1): 62–71

Maruyama T C 1999 Hospice care and culture: a comparison of the hospice movement in the west and Japan. Ashgate, Brookfield, VT

Rosenberger N R (ed) 1992 Japanese sense of self. Cambridge University Press, New York

Smith R J 1999 The living and the dead in Japanese popular religion. In: Long S O (ed) Lives in motion: composing circles of self and community in Japan. (East Asia Series) Cornell University, Ithaca, NY

Tanida N 1997 The social acceptance of euthanasia does not stem from patients' autonomy in Japan. Eubios Journal of Asian and International Bioethics 7 (2): 43–46

World Health Organization 2001 Educational module on female genital mutilation. WHO, Geneva

11

Using the human rights paradigm in health ethics: the problems and the possibilities*

Wendy Austin

Human rights may be the most globalised political value of our time. The rights paradigm has been criticised, however, for being theoretically unsound, legalistic, individualistic and based on assumptions that cannot be sustained. Wendy Austin considers here the problems and the possibilities of a rights approach in addressing health ethics issues. The practical example she uses shows that in ethics many people and agencies need to work together, and therefore that ethics concerns every person and is as much about responsibility as about rights.

INTRODUCTION

Human rights may be the most globalized political value of our times,[1] a new world ideology. As well as legal norms, human rights serve as the moral underpinnings of contemporary international relations, setting the individual at the core of national and international concerns.[2,3] Rights are set out in normative instruments that give recognition to the dignity and respect of every person. The rights paradigm, however, is not without its critics: legalistic, individualistic and based on the assumption that there is a given and universal humanness, it arises from a western ethos that sits rather uneasily in the East. Rights have rhetorical force and violations are imbued with shame, but their real efficacy can be questioned.

The use of the human rights paradigm in the

area of health ethics is relatively new. Proponents point to its power to frame health as an entitlement rather than a commodity. This has substantive implications for the content and processes of health ethics. The problems and the possibilities of employing a rights approach in addressing health ethics issues are explored in this article.

THE HUMAN RIGHTS PARADIGM

The central assumption of the rights paradigm is that every person can make certain claims based solely on their humanness. This idea of 'natural rights' or the 'rights of man' arose in struggles for equality and freedom. Britain's Magna Carta of 1215 is recognized as one of the earliest rights documents.[4] John Locke used rights language to underpin his philosophical argument against the divine right of kings, arguing that all people are creatures of the same species born to the same advantages of nature, with equal entitlement to natural freedoms.[5] American and French revolutionaries used natural rights to assert liberty from their respective kings, later securing these 'natural, inalienable, and sacred'[6] rights in constitutional documents. Thomas Paine wrote in *Rights of man*:

Natural rights are those which appertain to man in right of his existence. Of this kind are all the intellectual rights, or rights of the mind, and also all those rights of acting as an individual for his own comfort and happiness, which are not injurious to the natural rights of others.

Civil rights, arising from membership in

* Reprinted from Nursing Ethics 2001; 8(13): 183–195, by kind permission of the publisher, Arnold, London.

society, have their foundation in these natural pre-existing rights.[7]

A human rights approach to securing justice and peace in the world was taken by the international community in the aftermath of World War II. Previously, international law governed only relations among nations. The recognition of Nazi war crimes as 'crimes against humanity' and sincere aspirations for a better world, free from fear and want, stimulated attempts to protect individuals. The first international proclamation of the rights and freedoms of all people was the Universal Declaration of Human Rights (UDHR),[8] adopted by the General Assembly of the United Nations (UN) on December 10, 1948. The UDHR makes the protection and fulfilment of individuals' rights, as defined in the charter, the responsibility of governments. It has led to: national human rights laws; international treatises on civil and political rights; economic, social and cultural rights; women's rights; children's rights; and rights of protection against racial discrimination.

Peoples' rights are about the rights of specific groups, as well as individuals. Women are, to date, the most successful group to delineate rights claims. The Convention on the Elimination of all Forms of Discrimination Against Women (in force since 1981) has 165 states party to it.[9] It affirms, together with gender equality, the reproductive rights of women. Violence against women as a rights violation has gained increasing recognition (e.g. in the 1993 Vienna Declaration and Programme of Action). The 1995 UN Conference on Women in Beijing identified the right of women to decide freely all matters related to their sexuality and child bearing and their need for access to financial credit, as well as declaring the systematic rape of women in war as a war crime. Other groups taking a rights approach to oppression are ethnic/racial groups (e.g. indigenous peoples), persons with lesbian or gay sexual orientation, and persons with disabilities. The rights of these collectives, however, are a contentious area of rights discourse, with many people being suspicious of the 'special interests' of particular social groups.[10]

Human rights are said to be in their third generation. O'Sullivan[11] refers to Vasak, a French jurist, who uses the norms of French revolution as descriptors of the phases. The first, *liberté*, consisted of civil and political rights. These are, in a sense, negative rights because many are rights to freedom from things like torture and arbitrary arrest. The second phase, *égalité*, focused on economic, social, and cultural rights. These tend to be positive rights, such as the right to safe and healthy working conditions. The third phase is in formation: *fraternité*, or solidarity, a response to the current domination of market-place values under economic globalization.

Knoppers, chair of the Ethics Committee of the Human Genome Project, puts a different slant on the third generation of rights; she names it 'bioethics'.[12] As evidence, she points to the power of biotechnology to change human existence and to a recent rights document, the Universal Declaration on the Human Genome and Human Rights, adopted by the United Nations Educational, Scientific and Cultural Organization in 1997 … In this document, human rights principles are applied to interventions affecting human genes, with emphasis placed on three points: the human genome as symbolically 'the heritage of humanity', the dignity of the human person, and the rejection of genetic reductionism. The protection of individuals and solidarity for vulnerable families and populations are addressed, but freedom for research development is particularly stressed.[13]

The interplay between a new phase focused on biotechnology as opposed to one geared to solidarity is noteworthy. Biotechnology is big business. Life forms can now be patented,[14] and questions, such as: 'Who owns genes and other pieces of DNA?' must soon be answered. This is a new aspect to an existing realization that a few powerful people may come to control the world's resources. A priority on civil and political rights would highlight their freedom to do so, while a focus on solidarity, placing greater value on economic, social and cultural rights, would highlight other things, such as the continuous improvement of living conditions for people around the globe. Whether a bioethics or a communitarian perspective comes to dominate the current phase, rights related to health will be an issue.

THE RIGHT TO HEALTH

Taken literally, a right to health makes little sense: no government can guarantee the health of a citizen. The right to health, however, is actually shorthand in rights discourse for the more complex terminology of international treatises and documents.[15] Health within the rights paradigm is an entitlement, a very different concept from health as a commodity. As a right, individuals can lay claim to it, which, symbolically at least, has great significance. Governments ratifying UN agreements with articles pertaining to health are obliged to report on actions taken to improve the health of their people.

In 1946 the international community, through the adoption of the World Health Organization's (WHO) Constitution, accepted as a fundamental right 'the enjoyment of the highest attainable standard of health'. Soon after, in 1948, article 25 of the UDHR[8] enshrined:

[everyone's] right to a standard of living adequate for the health and well-being of himself and his family, including food, clothing, housing, and medical care and necessary social services, and the right to security in the event of unemployment, sickness, disability, widowhood, old age, or other lack of livelihood in circumstances beyond his control.

Since then, rights relating to health have been included in many international rights documents:

* Universal Declaration of Human Rights, article 25
* International Covenant on Economic, Social and Cultural Rights, article 12
* Optional Protocol to the International Covenant on Civil and Political Rights
* Second Optional Protocol aimed at the Abolition of the Death Penalty
* International Convention on the Elimination of all Forms of Racial Discrimination
* Convention on the Elimination of all Forms of Discrimination Against Women
* Convention on the Rights of the Child
* Convention Against Torture and Other Cruel, Inhuman or Degrading Treatment or Punishment
* International Convention on the Protection of the Rights of all Migrant Workers and Members of their Families (not entered into force as yet)
* UN Resolution 46/119: Protection of Persons with Mental Illness and Improvement of Mental Health Care
* World Health Organization Constitution

Health as a universal human right means equal opportunity of access to quality health care, regardless of gender, race, social, economic and geographical facts. Mahler, a former Director General of WHO, says that the central issue for health is the ethical basis of health development.[16] This means that health matters must be considered in the broadest social context, with the impact of powerful economic and political forces that affect the health of peoples acknowledged.[17] Justice is a crucial issue in the rights paradigm.

POSSIBILITIES OF A HUMAN RIGHTS AND HEALTH LINK

A link between health and human rights may allow us to meet global health challenges in a better way. Jonathan Mann, a key contributor in this area, conceptualized the relationship between health and human rights as two continuums: a horizontal one with medicine and public health at opposing ends, and a vertical one with the ends being ethics and human rights. Mann believed that ethics was most useful to medicine and human rights to public health.[18] This, however, seems a rather awkward concept. Medicine, public health, ethics and rights are more related and integrated than this would indicate. Dick Sobsey argues that the artificial separation between bioethics and human rights has allowed bioethicists to function in the artificial environment of the medical setting, ignoring the far-reaching implications of some of their ideas.[19] Although the relationship between ethics and rights needs further elucidation, some links between health and human rights have been delineated.

Impact of health policies and practices on human rights

Gro Harlem Brundtland, Director General of WHO, acknowledges that: 'By design, neglect or ignorance, health policies and programs can promote and protect or conversely restrict or violate human rights (p. 23).[20] Human rights violations can be inherent in the design and implementation of health policies. For example, strategies for infectious disease control have often infringed upon rights in such ways as mandatory testing and quarantine/isolation. These infringements were justified in the name of the public good.[21] The integration of human rights concerns with health care strategies is, however, modifying such approaches. When WHO responded to the AIDS pandemic, it fostered a new attitude. Recognizing the serious threat of discrimination against persons with HIV/AIDS, WHO addressed the protection of their rights in the Global Aids Strategy, a first in the history of epidemic control.[22]

Discriminatory practices against ethnic, religious and racial groups (including denial of access to care or the giving of inferior care) still compromises the health of many. Discrimination can occur in extreme forms, such as ethnic cleansing and genocide. It can also occur when there is a failure to acknowledge the health problems of particular groups or when the barriers to the access of health services are ignored. Under apartheid in South Africa, for example, health care was fragmented for segregationist purposes and differed enormously by race, even though this contravened medical ethics.[23,24] The other health rights issues are: lack of attention to health hazards creating dangerous environments; unethical research practices putting vulnerable populations at risk[25]; and failure to respect the dignity of persons with disabilities.

A Human Rights Impact Assessment tool has been developed to help to evaluate the effect of public health policies on human dignity and rights. Evolving from work at the Harvard School of Public Health, it draws upon their experience with policies for infectious diseases. The tool takes policy makers through such steps as 'Clarify the public health purpose' and 'If a coercive measure is truly necessary to avert a significant risk, guarantee fair procedures to persons affected.'[26] Its use is one way to sensitize health care policy makers to human rights issues.

Health impacts of human rights violations

Extreme poverty, trafficking in persons, and the protection of minorities [were] the urgent rights issues identified for the year 2000 by the UN's Office of the High Commissioner for Human Rights. The potential for negative impact on the health of those involved seems obvious. The profoundly poor lack even the basics of a healthy life: sufficient water and food, rest, clothes, shelter … hope. People treated as a commodity in a transnational industry that sells or coerces them into a life of exploitation and slavery are put both physically and mentally at grave risk, as are members of oppressed minority groups who experience torture, rape and imprisonment under inhumane conditions. Entire communities are affected by such rights violations and their significant and long-term impact on health.

Other pervasive rights violations also impact negatively on health. Violation of the right to information can mean that individuals are unaware of the harmful effects of tobacco or of ways to prevent sexually transmitted infection. Violation of the right to just and favourable work conditions can lead to death and disability. Denial of education, in particular to women, severely limits the ability to choose and support healthier life styles and to provide a healthy childhood for one's offspring.[21] Human rights are deemed essential for every human's well-being, so it can be said that any contravention will have health-related consequences.

Health professionals and human rights protection and violation

The Doctors' Trial in Nuremberg in 1946–1947 revealed extreme examples of physicians violating human rights, including the right to life. This shocked the world, but in fact there is a history of physicians participating in state or church sanctioned torture.[27] Despite clear exhortations to the contrary (e.g. the UN resolution on the principles of medical ethics relevant to health personnel in the protection of prisoners (1982); the ICN's position statement on nurses' role in protecting human rights (1983, adopted 1998) … and in the care/protection of prisoners/detainees (1989, adopted 1998), physicians and other health professionals continue today to participate in torture. They do so in such ways as examining detainees prior to torture, monitoring torture to prevent death, and reviving victims for further torture, taking part in torture, such as the misuse of psychotropic medications, the development of techniques of torture, falsifying medical information, and remaining silent about torture.[28] Most recently, a news report claimed that 'Medical experts advised IRA on ways to shoot victims without killing them.'[29] Professional groups are working to expose such perversion of expertise. An excellent perspective on the difficulties involved may be found in an article by Brennan and Kirschner; they describe an inquiry after the Gulf War by Physicians for Human Rights into allegations of rights violations in Kuwait.[30]

Health professionals can protect rights by identifying, documenting and testifying about the violation of rights (e.g. occupational health violations). They can promote health rights by: providing scientific information about public health problems; helping the public to monitor and question health systems; influencing policies by taking positions and mobilizing support from their professional groups; and educating themselves about human rights.[21,31,32] Groups such as Physicians for Human Rights and Global Lawyers and Physicians exist to help professionals to collaborate in protecting such rights.

Health practitioners can suffer for fulfilling their roles without discrimination concerning the ethnic, racial or political identity of patients. Incidents such as the 1996 shooting of six delegates (including five nurses) of the International Red Cross in Novye Atagi in Chechnya, and the killing of nurses providing hospital care to Burundian soldiers in Zaire, are terrible reminders of this. In 2000, for the third time, the ICN joined with the International Pharmaceutical Federation and the World Medical Association to request a UN special rapporteur to monitor and ensure the independence and integrity of health professionals.[33] There are also efforts being made towards the establishment of an international medical tribunal that could articulate and enforce stands on medical ethics and human rights.[34]

PROBLEMS WITH THE HUMAN RIGHTS PARADIGM

The human rights paradigm can be used to frame efforts to improve the health status of the world's population, but should it be? There are criticisms of the paradigm that need to be considered, some of which have existed since the idea of natural rights was first conceived. They include arguments that rights are theoretically unsound, legalistic, individualistic and based on the assumption that there is a given and universal humanness. A brief overview of these critiques follows.

The nonsense critique

The human rights paradigm lacks a sound theoretical basis and is conceptually flawed. Proponents may describe rights as *a priori*, given naturally as a part of human existence, but this is not a sensible argument. It is a tautology and devoid of meaning. The utilitarian, Jeremy Bentham, in the eighteenth century, denounced rights as coming not from nature, but 'from a hard heart operating upon a cloudy mind'. 'Natural rights is simple nonsense', he said, 'natural and imprescriptible rights, rhetorical nonsense – nonsense upon stilts.' There may be reasons for wishing that rights existed, he admitted, but 'Want is not supply. Hunger is not bread' (p. 53).[35] The only strength he found in the argument for rights was in the lungs of those who used it.

The 'nonsense' stance is maintained today. For instance, from a very different referent than Bentham, Phra Dhammapidok, a prominent Thai Buddhist scholar, also criticizes human rights as being pure invention, so lacking a firm and lasting foundation of truth.[36] Rights, it can be cogently argued, are artificial, political values created by human decisions, not a mysterious condition of humanity.[37]

Is this a real problem? Does the lack of an epistemological foundation for human rights matter to anyone outside philosophers? Wilson, for one, argues in the affirmative: 'Rights without a meta-narrative are like a car without seat-belts; on hitting the first moral bump with ontological implications, the passengers' safety is jeopardized (p. 8).'[38] Some, however, suggest that concerns about rights theory are little more than distractions. What matters is that the human rights paradigm is a powerful tool for upholding human dignity and combating human suffering. Its theoretical foundations may always be problematic but, in practice, the rights paradigm has meaning.[39] Natural or contrived, there is a validity to rights that ordinary people around the world understand and embrace. Albert Einstein put it this way: 'The existence and validity of human rights are not written in the stars… [They] have been conceived and taught by enlightened individuals in the course of history.'[40]

The legislative critique

Rights are forensic.[41] Although human rights are conceived as existing before any laws, it is legislation that is used to enshrine and protect them. This can be problematic if the infrastructures to support legal solutions are not in place. Critics point out that effective international legal mechanisms to enforce human rights are still to be realized.

The International Court of Justice and Human Rights is the judicial organ of the UN but, as the international covenants on human rights do not specifically provide for adjudication by the Court, few cases concerning rights have been heard. Individuals and nongovernmental organizations cannot be parties in litigation before this Court. Optional protocols, however, have been designed for some human rights conventions (e.g. the International Covenant on Civil and Political Rights). These allow individuals or groups to submit claims if the accused state is a signatory of the protocol. Past decisions have achieved results, with prisoners being released and compensation being paid to victims. Optional protocols were adopted recently to the Convention on the Rights of the Child[42] regarding the involvement of children in armed conflict, and the sale, prostitution and pornographic use of children. A new permanent International Criminal Court (ICC) is coming into existence to address gross rights violations: genocide, war crimes and crimes against humanity. […]

Mary Robinson, the UN High Commissioner for Human Rights, points to such developments as the ICC as evidence that real and practical progress is being made. Nevertheless, she acknowledges that the horrors that led to the creation of the UDHR still exist.[43] Overall, there is frustration that, despite the courts and all the rights agreements, rights can be openly abused with impunity: '[W]hy are there all these human rights standards but the bodies keep piling up (p. 2)?[44] Sanctions have rarely been applied against, for instance, nations who persistently ignore their obligation to ensure basic health care for all.[45] Globalization is only increasing the problem: it is multinational corporations and banks that are actually setting policies and political agendas.[46,47]

It may be that a legalistic approach can never make a significant difference. Evans and Hancock argue that it actually limits the means to address abuses. Efforts that could make a real difference, like determining the political, social and economic reasons why rights are violated, are not within its scope. These authors are of the opinion that rights give us the illusion of doing something without doing anything, an illusory solution that is worse than no solution at all.[48]

The individualistic critique

The individual is foremost in the human rights paradigm. This has been construed as placing persons in opposition to their community, as constructing a narrow and negative perspective of the individual's relationship to society.[35] Marx, for instance, contended that rights arguments presuppose conflict between isolated individuals and this symbolized for him the alienation of the human from 'species being'.[49] Hegel found that a rights approach lacked any substantial basis for an ethical way of life, that it offered nothing over and above individualism.[50] The privileging of the individual before the group does not fit many cultures outside the West. The ethos of Asian societies, for instance, tends to put community needs before personal freedom.

Rebuttals of such critiques acknowledge that rights are claims for the equal entitlements of individual people. It is refuted, however, that this excludes support for the moral solidarity of all human beings. It is argued that rights are about 'community': they delineate the conditions necessary for people to have dignified and flourishing lives within their communities. Hyudai Sakamoto, the founder of the Japanese Bioethics society, pushes the idea of community further in relation to rights. In postulating a global bioethic, he calls for a minimization of *human* rights, arguing from a traditional Asian perspective that human beings are not separate and distinct from nature and other living things. Their rights should not predominate in a true global context.[51]

The relativistic critique

There can be no universal human rights because we do not have a universal human community.[52] This argument, grounded in traditional anthropology, presupposes that no common humanity exists, that human nature is strictly a product of history and culture. Within this relativist position, it is maintained that moral values arise within particular cultural communities and that these values cannot be judged by outsiders. Traditional and local majority values must trump, not essentialist rights.[53]

This position is challenged by the observation that there are at least some elements that all human beings share (e.g. mortality; bodily capacities, like hunger, pain, sexual desire; cognitive abilities; capacity for affiliation with others). Whatever our culture, we are not so radically different that we cannot be identified as members of the same species, with similar basic needs.[54] Furthermore, human rights do not mean cultural imperialism and the subversion of traditional loyalties. They are, however, protection for the individual against the public violence or stigmatization that can be used to enforce traditional and communal bonds.[55]

Can the rights paradigm be authentically supported by normative traditions outside western democratic ideals? This remains under debate. Within the Buddhist community, for instance, some find human rights in tune with the ideals of classical Buddhism, with differences of form, not substance. Other Buddhist scholars fundamentally disagree.[36,56,57] It may be that rights are not so western after all. The first rights document is probably the 2500-year-old, Persian Charter of Cyrus, which protected liberty, security, freedom of movement, the right to own property and certain economic and social rights.[58]

A comparison of human rights charters across regions indicates that both common elements and regional characteristics exist. All charters include protection of life and liberty as the most basic right; all include the right to protection from torture, inhuman or degrading treatment, the liberty of the person and the right to a fair trial. The African charter does not include a right to privacy and family life, as American and European charters do, but a duty of the State to assist the family as the custodian of community morals and traditional values is named. The American charter includes freedom of expression and prohibits censorship. An interesting question arose during this review, concerning how 'region' should be defined? Neighbours may be more dissimilar in values that distant nations.[11]

Societies may interpret, prioritize and realize values differently, but it does seem possible to reach consensus on some universals. Pluralist universalism is the term that Parekh gives to this. He argues that an open-minded, cross-cultural dialogue will allow us to determine which rights we can all respect.[59]

A CASE EXAMPLE

The human rights paradigm brings both possibilities and problems. In order to consider them in context, it may be helpful to examine how a rights approach to a health problem can be enacted. A case illustrating a human rights approach to access to clean drinking water, published in *Health and Human Rights*, provides an example.[60]

Certain villages in Israel, populated by Bedouin Arabs, were unrecognized by the State and thus were not connected to the national water network. The villagers lacked sufficient quantity and quality of water and experienced outbreaks of disease, such as hepatitis A, because of contaminated water supplies. Petitions to the Government failed. Access to safe drinking water for these communities was achieved, however, when a public health physician, a nurse, an environmental engineer and a human rights lawyer took the villages' case before the International Water Tribunal (IWT), an independent forum for adjudicating water issues.

Trusted by village leaders, these professionals formed a team to gather evidence and prepare a brief, which took one year. The physician and the nurse compiled health statistics; the engineer reported on the quantity and quality of the village water. The nurse researched the cause of the hepatitis A outbreak and linked it to contaminated water. She surveyed incidences of diarrhoeal disease in children less than five years of age. When the case went to the IWT in 1992, the tribunal found insufficient evidence to show discrimination between Arabs and Jews, but also found insufficient evidence that public interest required nonrecognition of these communities (the Israeli government's argument). The denial of water was deplored, however, and the IWT recommended connection of the villages to the national water network, as well as co-operation among those affected in finding equitable solutions to planning and zoning. The case received major press coverage and became an issue in the Israeli elections. The new government connected all unrecognized villages to the water network.

This case does illuminate the potential and the limitations of the human rights paradigm in relation to fostering health. The people of the villages had to become involved in finding a solution. The brief required expertise, diligence, time and teamwork. Facts and scientific evidence were necessary to support their position. There had to be a place to which to take the case. In this instance ,there was – a tribunal with no power to enforce its decisions, but which, nevertheless, had moral, if not legal, force. The stigma of rights violations meant that shame became a tool, with the news media playing a crucial role in putting the information before the public. The public, in turn, had to respond and use political pressure to instigate change.

CONCLUSION

The human rights paradigm can, and is, being used to make a difference in the health of individuals and communities. Despite substantial criticisms, it offers a new way to consider issues in health ethics. Conceptualizing health as a right calls attention to health as a social good rather than as a strictly medical problem. It reminds policy makers that, whenever the rights of individuals are limited in the name of the public good, those limitations must be scrutinized. It keeps before us not only the principles of human dignity and equality but also the obligations we have to one another.[15] These seem necessary perspectives for the health of a global community.

To utilize the rights paradigm, health professionals will need to understand its strengths and weaknesses. They will need to ensure that students in health disciplines are educated about the relationship between health and human rights, about the health consequences of rights violations, about the impact of health policy on human rights, and about their own accountability. They will need actively to envision a world in which all persons have an equal opportunity to live in dignity with a chance for a healthy life.

Acknowledgement

This work was supported by a research fellowship from the Alberta Heritage Foundation for Medical Research.

REFERENCES

1 Wilson R ed. Human rights: culture and context. London: Pluto Press, 1997
2 Follow-up to the World Conference on Human Rights, Report of the United Nations High Commissioner for Human Rights, September 11, 1998; A/53/372. New York: UN.
3 Sumner LW. Rights. In: LaFollette H ed. The Blackwell guide to ethical theory. Oxford: Blackwell, 2000: 288–305.
4 Brown C. Universal human rights: a critique. In: Dunne T, Wheeler NJ eds. Human rights in global politics. Cambridge: Cambridge University Press, 1999: 103–27.
5 Locke J. Two treatises of government. Laslett P ed. Cambridge: Cambridge University Press, 1960. (Original published 1689.)
6 Declaration of the Rights of Man and the Citizen, 1789; later prefixed to the 1791 French Constitution.
7 Paine T. Rights of man. Ware: Wordsworth Editions, 1996. (First published 1790–1791.)
8 United Nations. Universal Declaration of Human Rights. Adopted and proclaimed by General Assembly resolution 217 A (III), 10 December 1948, New York: UN.
9 United Nations. Convention on the Elimination of all Forms of Discrimination Against Women. Adopted and opened for signature, ratification and accession by General Assembly resolution 34/80 of 18 December 1979, New York: UN.
10 Felice W. Taking suffering seriously: the importance of collective human rights. Albany, NY: State University of New York Press; 1996.
11 O'Sullivan D. The history of relativism. Int J Hum Rights 1998; 2(3): 22–48
12 Knoppers B. Human rights and genomics. In: Bhatia GS, O'Neill JS, Gall GL, Bendin PD eds. Peace, justice and freedom: human rights challenges for the new millennium. Edmonton: University of Alberta Press, 2000: 259–65.
13 United Nations Educational, Scientific and Cultural Organization. Universal Declaration on the Human Genome and Human Rights. Adopted by the General Conference of UNESCO, 11 November 1997. Available at: http://www.unesco.org/opi/29gencon
14 Spears T. Mouse decision will open the floodgates: biotech firms say patents allow them to protect investments, and the ruling is the green light they've been waiting for. Edmonton Journal 2000 Aug 4; Sect A: 13.
15 Leary V. The right to health in international human rights law. Health Hum Rights 1994; 1(l): 24–56.
16 Mahler H. The challenge of global health: how can we do better? Health Hum Rights 1997; 2(3): 71–75.
17 Benetar S. The biotechnology era: a story of two lives. In: Bhatia GS, O'Neill JS, Gall CL, Bendin PD eds. Peace, justice and freedom: human rights challenges for the new millennium. Edmonton: University of Alberta Press, 2000: 237–43.
18 Mann JM. Medicine and public health, ethics and human rights. In: Mann JM, Gruskin S, Grodin MA, Annas C eds. Health and human rights: a reader. New York: Routiedge, 1999: 439–52.
19 Sobsey D. Human rights, bioethics and disability. In: Bhatia GS, O'Neill JS, Gall GL, Bendin PD eds. Peace, justice and freedom: human rights challenges for the new millennium. Edmonton: University of Alberta Press, 2000: 237–43.
20 Brundtland GH. Fifty years of synergy between health and rights. Health Hum Rights 1998; 3(2): 21–25.
21 Mann JM, Gostin L, Gruskin S, Brennan T, Lazzarini Z, Fineberg H. Health and human rights. In: Mann IM, Gruskin S, Grodin MA, Annas G. Health and human rights: a reader. New York: Routledge, 1999: 7–20.
22 Gruskin S, Mann J, Tarantola D. Past, present and future: AIDS and human rights. Health Hum Rights 1997; 2(4): 1–3.
23 Nightingale E, Hannibal K, Geiger J, Hartmann, L, Lawrence R, Spurlock J. Apartheid medicine: health and human rights in South Africa. JAMA 1990; 264: 2097–102.
24 Bloche MC. Apartheid medicine and its moral aftermath. Proceedings of the XXVth Anniversary Congress on Law and Mental Health; 2000 July 10; Siena, Italy: 98.
25 Writing Group for the Consortium for Health and Human Rights. Commentaries: health and human rights. JAMA 1998; 280: 462–64.
26 Gostin L, Mann J. Towards the development of a human rights impact assessment for the formulation and evaluation of public health policies. Health Hum Rights 1994; 1(l): 59–80.
27 Wenzel T, Zoghlami A. The dark side of medicine and healing. Proceedings of the XXVth Anniversary Congress on Law and Mental Health; 2000 July 10; Siena, Italy: 98–99.
28 Nightingale E. The role of physicians in human rights. Law Med Health Care 1990; 18: 132–39.
29 Brogan B, Daily Telegraph, London. In: Edmonton Journal 2000 June 16; Sect A:5.
30 Brennan T, Kirschner R. Medical ethics and human rights violations: the Iraqui occupation of Kuwait and its

aftermath. Ann Intern Med 1992; 117: 78–82.

31 Hannibal K, Lawrence R. The health professional as human rights promoter: ten years of Physicians for Human Rights (USA). Health Hum Rights 1996; 2(l): 111–27.

32 Moore K, Randolph K, Toubia N, Kirberger E The synergistic relationship between health and human rights: a case study using female genital mutilation. Health Hum Rights 1997; 2(2): 137–46.

33 International Council of Nurses: press release. Nurses, pharmacists and doctors call for a UN special rapporteur to monitor the protection and independence of health professionals. Geneva: ICN, 10 Apr 2000.

34 Annas G, Grodin M. Medicine and human rights: reflections on the fiftieth anniversary of the Doctors' Trial. Health Hum Rights 1996; 2(l): 6–21.

35 Waldron J. 'Nonsense upon stilts:' Bentham, Burke and Marx on the rights of man. London: Methuen, 1987.

36 Hongladarom S. Buddism and human rights in the thoughts of Sulak Sivaraksa and Phra Dhammapidok. J Buddhist Ethics Online Conference on Buddhism and Human Rights; 1995 Oct 1–14; 1–12. Available at: http://jbe.1a.psu.edu/1995conf/honglada.txt

37 MacDonald M. Natural rights. In: Waldron J ed. Theories of rights. Oxford: Oxford University Press, 1984: 21–40.

38 Wilson RA. Human rights, culture and context: an introduction. In: Wilson RA ed. Human rights, culture and context. London: Pluto Press, 1997: 1–27.

39 Hurrell A. Power, principles and prudence: protecting human rights in a deeply divided world. In: Dunne T, Wheeler NJ eds. Human rights in global politics. Cambridge: Cambridge University Press, 1999: 277–302.

40 French AP ed. Einstein: a centenary volume. Cambridge, MA: Harvard University Press, 1979: 305–306.

41 Midgley M. Transnational civil society. In: Dunne T, Wheeler NJ eds. Human rights in global politics. Cambridge UK: Cambridge University Press, 1999: 161–74.

42 United Nations High Commissioner for Human Rights. Declaration on the Rights of the Child. Proclaimed by General Assembly resolution 1386 (XIV) 20 November 1989, New York, UN.

43 Robinson M. The challenge of the future for human rights. In: Bhatia CS, O'Neill IS, Gall GL, Bendin PD eds. Peace, justice and freedom: human rights challenges for the new millennium. Edmonton: University of Alberta Press, 2000; 11–13.

44 Dunne T, Wheeler N. Introduction. In: Dunne T, Wheeler N eds. Human rights in global politics. New York: Cambridge University Press, 1999: 1–28.

45 Kirby M. The right to health fifty years on: still sceptical? Health Hum Rights 1999; 4(l): 6–25.

46 Freidman T. The Lexus and the olive tree. New York: Farrar Straus Giroux, 1999.

47 Ohmae K. The borderless world. New York: Harper Perennial, 1990.

48 Evans T, Hancock E. Doing something without doing anything: international human rights law and the challenge of globalisation. Int J Hum Rights 1998; 2(3): 1–21.

49 Marx KH. On the Jewish question. (Written in 1843.) Text available at: http://csf.colorado.edu/mirrors/marxists.org/reference /archive/hegel/marx/kmjewish.htm

50 Hegel GW. Hegel's philosophy of right. (Knox TM, trans.) Oxford: Clarendon Press, 1964.

51 Sakamoto H. A new possibility of global bioethics as an intercultural social tuning technology. Unpublished paper presented at Health Ethics: a Global Context, preconference to the 11th Annual Canadian Bioethies Conference; 1999 Oct 27; Edmonton, Canada.

52 Booth K. Three tyrannies. In: Dunne T, Wheeler N eds. Human rights in global politics. New York: Cambridge University Press, 1999: 31–70.

53 James S. Recognizing international human rights and cultural relativism: the case of female circumcision. Bioethics 1994; 8(l): 1–26.

54 Nussbaum M. Human capabilities, female human beings. In: Nussbaum M, Glover J eds. Women, culture and development: a study of human capabilities. Oxford: Clarendon Press, 1995: 61–104.

55 Lindholm T. The emergence and development of human rights: an interpretation with a view to cross-cultural and interreligious dialogue. Unpublished article presented at the Diyarbakir International Conference on Human Rights; 1997 Sep 26–28; Diyarbakir, Turkey.

56 Keown D. Are there human rights in Buddhism? J Buddhist Ethics Online Conference on Buddhism and Human Rights; 1995. Oct 1–14: 1–18. Available at: http://jbe.1a.psu.edu/2/keown2.html

57 Junger PD. Why the Buddha has no rights. J Buddhist Ethics Online Conference on Buddhism and Human Rights 1995 Oct 1–14. Available at: http://jbe.1a.psu.edu/2/jungerhtml

58 Milne A. Human rights and the diversity of morals: a philosophical analysis of rights and obligations in the global system. In: Wright M ed. Rights and obligations in North-South relations. Toronto: Macmillan, 1986: 8–33.

59 Parekh B. Non-enthnocentric universalism. In: Dunne T, Wheeler NJ eds. Human rights in global politics. Cambridge: Cambridge University Press, 1999: 128–59.

60 Kanaaneh H, McKay F, Sims E. A human rights approach for access to clean drinking water: a case study. Health Hum Rights 1995; 1(2): 190–204.

12

Socratic dialogue: an example

Stan van Hooft

This and the next chapter deal with a tool for understanding and learning ethics rather than a specific approach to the subject. Socratic dialogue is an increasingly useful instrument for learning in depth about a particular subject, perhaps one that is difficult or intricate. In this chapter Stan van Hooft gives an account of one such dialogue that he had facilitated. At one level of reading this chapter, it was not a successful dialogue because the question it was meant to answer—Why does caring matter in nursing?—never received a satisfactory answer. However, at what Stan describes as the 'metadialogue', a great deal was addressed and discussed. The metadialogue is as important as the more obvious dialogue and, indeed, what is learned here throws considerable light on the basic question, although not from the obvious angle. A skilled facilitator can interpret the different levels for the group gathered for the dialogue. Here, it is the facilitator who writes about the dialogue and, in the self-analysis taking place in this chapter, an important aspect of ethics is highlighted: listening, hearing what is said, honestly understanding, and that all learning is important, however it happens.

PROLOGUE

Margaret was about 22 years old and a nurse not long out of training when she was assigned to a military hospital in an outlying suburb of a major American city. The Vietnam War was raging and soldiers were being flown in directly from jungle field hospitals. While on duty in the early hours of one morning she was called upon to attend to a newly arrived marine. It would be a confrontation that was to have a profound effect on her. Peter, who was about the same age as Margaret, had had both his legs blown off in a mine explosion some days earlier and had lost his right arm up to and including his shoulder. His wounds had been stabilised and the blood flow stopped, but what was needed now was a change of dressing and the application of antiseptic and soothing ointments. Margaret baulked at the shoulder. She would have to place her hand right into the open socket close by Peter's head. She would not be able to avoid his gaze and, perhaps, she would not be able to mask her revulsion and pity at such a horrible wound.

Margaret steeled herself. She had never had to do anything so difficult. Although Peter was not in much pain, she felt the enormity of his loss and the tragedy of his trauma, and could do nothing more than focus on her task and on the gentleness of her touch upon the ghastly flesh before her. Peter's face was expressionless but his eyes gazed intently into Margaret's as she worked close to his face. He was to tell her some weeks later as he convalesced in the hospital that he had been watching to see if she would be repulsed by him. He said then that he had been immensely relieved at her air of acceptance during this first encounter. She had seemed to him not to be rejecting him for his shattered body. In this first encounter with a woman since the devastation of his virility he had been reassured of his value.

During the eight weeks that Margaret cared for Peter and came to know him, she could not help but think that he had given her more credit for this reaction than she deserved. It had been all she could do not to flee from his bedside. It had been hard to maintain the appearance of caring and even to hold her hand steady as she applied the ointment; and, yet, as a caring encounter, it had been a success and it had been important to them both.

THE METHOD OF SOCRATIC DIALOGUE

These events occurred some 30 years ago. The story was offered by Margaret as an example in a 'Socratic dialogue' that I facilitated recently with a group of nurses on the question: 'Why does caring matter in nursing?' Examples of this kind are central to the Socratic dialogue method. (It is for this reason that I sometimes call them 'real case Socratic dialogues' to distinguish them from other methods of personal interaction, group centred inquiry, or pedagogy, which use question and answer techniques reminiscent of the historical Socrates.)

A real case Socratic dialogue seeks to answer a general question. Examples of such questions that may be relevant in the field of nursing could be:

- What is human dignity?
- What is the meaning of suffering in our lives?
- How should we think about death?
- What is professional commitment?
- What should be my relation to patients?
- When should I give up?

Because such questions are too broad to generate a focused discussion, a dialogue begins with several examples relating to the question being offered by members of the group. These examples have to arise from the actual experience of participants and should relate a specific incident in which the matter of the question is at issue. The second step in the highly structured method of the dialogue is to discuss these examples briefly with a view to choosing just one on which to focus. The choice is made on the basis that the example will help the group to answer the dialogue question. Accordingly, even choosing the example already begins to uncover assumptions about the question and views about the answer with which the group is working. The purpose of beginning a dialogue with examples from real life is to ground the discussion in reality and to avoid an over-intellectualised or abstract approach. Although one might expect that most nurses would have a view about why caring matters in nursing, it is best initially if these views are expressed by offering and analysing real-life cases rather than engaging in a purely theoretical discourse. Moreover, since the goal of the dialogue process is to achieve consensus, it helps to ground the discussion in concrete cases. People disagree on conceptual issues more often on the basis of different abstract theories rather than on the basis of their perception of real cases.

Having chosen an example, the third phase of the dialogue format requires the group to explore the example thoroughly and to ask the person who offered it as many questions as are necessary for them to have a deep understanding of it. Each participant must seek to understand the example to the extent that they can place themselves in it, as if they were in the shoes of the person who offered it. In the case before us, Margaret offered her story as an example of how caring matters in nursing. The group needs to position itself in Margaret's point of view so that group members can come to see why she thinks that caring mattered in this incident. In order to do this, they need to explore the example and to listen carefully to what Margaret says about it.

The fourth phase of the dialogue is to ask why the example is, indeed, an example that is relevant to the question. Given that the question for this dialogue was 'Why does caring matter in nursing?' this requirement could be met by asking whether the example was really an example of caring. In what way was Margaret's action a caring one? It could also be met by asking how caring mattered in this particular case. What difference did the caring quality of Margaret's action make? Given that the group has explored the example thoroughly, it needs no longer be just Margaret whose view on this is authoritative. Everyone can now 'own' the example and propose an answer to these questions from their own point of view, as they imagine themselves in Margaret's situation.

Once the group has answered the questions about why caring mattered in this particular case to its own satisfaction and agreement, it can then proceed to the final phase of the dialogue process. This fifth phase involves generalising from what has been discovered while focusing on the particular example, to develop a more general and theoretical answer to the question in its initial and general form. Such an answer would ideally apply to all cases of caring. In some dialogues, if there is time, the facilitator may even test the agreed-upon answer to the question by seeing whether it throws light on the examples that had been offered but not chosen by the group.

It is important for participants in the dialogue to stick to the chosen example during the third and fourth phases of the discussion. Introducing other examples or changing the one that had been chosen can serve only to confuse the dialogue. Moreover, participants should refrain, as far as possible, from being too theoretical and introducing ideas from books and abstract conceptual schemes. Although some level of theoretical understanding is important, it is essential that one's contributions to the discussion be grounded in the example and in one's own experiences of life as they relate to the example. It is important that each participant listens carefully to what others are saying in order to be able to respond to that. It often happens in other forms of discussion that one is thinking of what one is going to say next while others are talking. This would be worse than discourtesy in a Socratic dialogue because such a dialogue seeks to develop a chain of thinking in which each link is a response to the link before it. There will be many points in the discussion when no one (including the facilitator) knows where the chain of ideas is leading and it is important to stay with the discussion where it is currently situated rather than seeking to anticipate its outcome or steering it in a particular direction. Every contribution is a gem

that must be held up to the light in order to explore all its facets.

Such exploration is, above all else, a strenuous intellectual exercise. It involves clarifying one's ideas, expressing them in a way that reduces the risk of misinterpretation, seeking to understand what others are saying in ways that preserve their insights, and ensuring that all suggestions follow logically from what are claimed to be their reasons. The dialogue process aims at understanding and at consensus. Understanding does not consist just in having a grasp of what another has said; it must be a grasp that is in accordance with what the other intended to say. This requires frequent cross-checking to ensure that interlocutors are not at cross-purposes. Consensus also requires not only that one seeks to understand the views of others but that one be prepared to review and revise one's own views. Even to understand fully one's own views with all their implications and ramifications can be difficult; to do so in a dialogue context can sometimes require honesty and flexibility as well as the intellectual skills of rationality and clear thought.

To structure this intellectual effort effectively requires a commitment of time, a group that is not too large, and the services of an appropriately trained facilitator. Six hours is the minimum time for an effective dialogue and many take place over a number of days. Groups should consist of no more than 10 and no less than about six people. The facilitator has to exercise a judicious blend of listening and prodding, with a willingness to allow the conversation to move in its own direction and at its own pace. The main tools that facilitators have at their disposal are flip-charts and marking pens. Apart from the steps described earlier, the structure of the dialogue is provided by the notes and questions that the facilitator writes on the flip-chart. One of the several strategies available to facilitators is that of asking the group collectively to formulate interim or final conclusions in such a way that every word is discussed and agreed to before the group moves on to any further issues. It is often the debate over one word that uncovers disagreement where, previously, participants had falsely supposed that they had all seen a particular issue in the same way.

This dialogue structure is called 'Socratic' not because it consists of a facilitator moving a group, by way of prods and questions, to a position that the facilitator already has in mind. Rather, it is called 'Socratic' because it is premised on Socrates' idea that many people have an implicit knowledge of values and concepts that they would find it difficult to articulate fully, and that this knowledge can become a more effective constituent of a well-lived life to the extent that they can articulate it and understand it rationally. If this view is correct, then 'real case Socratic dialogue' can be a powerful instrument for developing virtue as well as for deepening knowledge.

THE DIALOGUE CONTINUES

Let us return now to the dialogue that I facilitated on the question: 'Why does caring matter in nursing?' The group has explored Margaret's example and the details in my narrative reconstruction of the example above have emerged. The question that the group should now explore is: 'Why did caring matter in this example?' However, as facilitator, I believed that the group was not clear on a question that was preliminary to this one, namely: 'In what did the caring consist in this example?'

In answer to this question, the following suggestions were made. Mandy said that Margaret's caring consisted in her seeming to know Peter and how he would feel when confronted by a woman while he was in his terribly reduced condition. Mandy thought that Margaret showed empathy with Peter's feelings. This idea was reiterated by Joan. She highlighted the empathic connection between Margaret and Peter and added that Margaret's giving of herself was unconditional. Feeling that this way of putting it seemed rather abstract or, perhaps, drawn from books rather than reflecting real experience, the group was keen to know what the nature of this 'unconditional giving of self' could be. How could it be described in terms that the group members would recognise from their own experience in the nursing setting and from their

exploration of Margaret's example? The best that the group was able to come up with in consideration of this idea was that Margaret had had to struggle within herself in order to prepare herself for the emotionally difficult procedure that she had to perform. Some members of the group were not satisfied, however, that this steeling of herself for the task was all that comprised 'unconditional self-giving'.

However, rather than proceed along this line of inquiry, the next contribution to the discussion introduced an entirely different thought. Gerry suggested that, in this example, as in any other, what caring consists of is whatever the person cared for says it is. In the example, caring is what Peter says it is. Peter had reported being encouraged by Margaret's apparent acceptance of him despite his injuries and so this constitutes caring. Gerry was pressed to explain her point. Did she think that anything at all that a recipient finds to be caring actually would be caring, no matter what was the attitude of the nurse? What role did Margaret's effort at controlling her feelings of revulsion play in constituting the act as one of caring? What role did her effort in softening and steadying her touch play in constituting the act as one of caring? Gerry refused to engage with these questions but simply insisted that caring was located somehow in Peter's response to Margaret.

It was Liz who now entered the discussion in order to try to overcome the impasse. She defined caring in the clinical setting as a patient's acknowledgement of an appropriate response on the part of the nurse to that patient's condition. Leaving aside that this definition was offered in the abstract rather than with reference to the example, the group asked why there should be such a stress on the patient rather than on the nurse. Why would caring be situated somehow in Peter's response rather than in Margaret's action or motivation? Gerry and Liz had an answer to this question, which clarified their position. They saw caring in holistic terms. An incidence of caring consists of many aspects, including the caring act and the recipient's response to it. The notion of caring refers to the whole nursing event and not just the nurse's contribution to it or her or his motivation for it. Caring resides in the whole episode. Peter and Margaret both participated in this caring event; their every gesture and glance, her touch and his receiving of it, her empathy and self-discipline, together with his need and vulnerability, are all constitutive of caring in the example. The more detail one adds to the story, the more one sees the caring. When asked what the caring would consist of then, or which features of the event differed from other features in that they constituted caring, Liz and Gerry offered this definition of caring: caring is a relatedness, a 'being in the moment' with the patient.

Without apparently noticing that this definition put the emphasis back on Margaret instead of Peter (or perhaps because it did so), everyone in the group seemed to be happy with this definition and with this account of caring in the example. On the other hand, as facilitator, I could not help but feel dissatisfied. To me it seemed too vague and it seemed that the group could not decide where to locate caring: in Peter, in Margaret, or in the relationship between them. After all, had not Margaret offered the example as one in which she had been the caring one, or had I just been assuming that? Even though the role of a facilitator does not extend to questioning a consensus reached by the group, I decided to probe further. Were the roles of carer and cared-for not different in a caring situation? Was it Margaret's delicate touch and sensitive behaviour that constituted the caring, or was it her determination not to display any revulsion towards the wounds? In what way does Peter's grateful receipt of the caring contribute to the whole story being one of caring?

Yet, probe as I would, the group was not willing to analyse the incident further or revise its definition. Indeed, my efforts to encourage a more analytical and clear probing of the relevant concepts were meeting with increasingly impatient resistance. Some in this all-female group accused me of engaging in the typically masculinist activity of seeking to impose a rational structure on an essentially emotional situation. The dialogue was beginning to evoke some feelings of disappointment and resentment on the part of some participants, and puzzlement and frustration on my part. It seemed time to enter into 'metadialogue'.

METADIALOGUE

The method of Socratic dialogue allows for the group to enter into a process of reflection and discussion on the dialogue process itself, at any point where this may be necessary. Any member of the group, as well as the facilitator, can call for a metadialogue and, when this happens, the group suspends its discussion and turns its attention to the dialogue process. Why is there a log jam? Why is a particular person not contributing? Does everyone understand where the discussion has gone? What strategies or questions could the group pursue in order to facilitate finding an answer to the dialogue question? On occasion, the group may even ask: Why is that participant being so d... annoying? With questions such as these, the group can review and re-order its discussion or uncover blockages that may be preventing progress.

On this occasion, it seemed to most of the group members that it was I myself, as facilitator, who was causing the problem. I was pressing the group to move into a rational, analytical direction that it felt no need to pursue. Certainly, Gerry and Liz thought that the group had achieved enough of an understanding of what caring was and that we could now proceed to the main dialogue question. Yet, how could we ask why caring matters in nursing if it was not even clear why it mattered in Margaret's story? This was not clear, because no one could agree where it was located in the example or what aspect of the example constituted the caring. Moreover, Liz was accusing me of being too much of a 'man', and not being sensitive to the holistic and more intuitive insights that the group had been developing. In my own defence I could say only that I was following the dialogue method as developed by the German philosopher Leonard Nelson (1882–1927), and developed by the Philosophical-Political Academy in Germany, the Society for the Furtherance of Critical Philosophy in the UK, and the Dutch Association for

Philosophical Practice (van Hooft 1999). Of course, this sounded too authoritarian and only inflamed the situation.

Perhaps it was the dialogue method itself that was the problem. It is certainly premised on the Enlightenment ideal of rationality, as well as on the Socratic idea that one does not really know something unless one can give a clear definition of it. The Enlightenment ideal of rationality suggests that anyone at all, irrespective of their background, nationality, race, class, abilities or gender, can agree with anyone else at all, provided only that everyone argues their case with impartiality, objectivity and fairness. This ideal further suggests that there really is a truth to be discovered about everything that matters, and that it is within the powers of human reason and human virtue to discover it. No disagreement is intractable because its source will always be found to be some ignorance, prejudice or blindness caused by irrationality or the unwillingness to adopt an impartial viewpoint. Leonard Nelson was inspired by the greatest of the Enlightenment philosophers, Kant, in developing the Socratic dialogue method precisely so that it would encapsulate the ideals of objectivity and be able to achieve such objective and consensual knowledge.

Further, in adopting the name of Socrates for his method, Nelson was expressing his conviction that Socratic dialogue would be a method for fulfilling that ancient nostrum, 'the unexamined life is not worth living'. How can one live by values that one does not understand? How can nurses dedicate their life to the professional practice of caring without having a clear grasp of what caring is? Although there will be many methods for achieving such clarity, Socratic dialogue certainly makes a strong claim to being an important technique for achieving such insight. The effort that is taken to define one's terms clearly and to reach consensus on the way that group members understand the key concepts in the discussion can result not only in greater clarity, but also in deeper convictions and stronger commitments; or so it is said.

Against this, Liz and Gerry in particular put forward what they described as a feminine ideal of knowledge. The bases of such knowledge are empathy and intuition. The model for such knowledge is not physical science or analytical philosophy but interpersonal rapport (Carper 1978). Central cases of such knowledge are the awareness that people have of one another in loving relationships. This knowledge does not improve in its quality to the degree that it is clearly defined, but to the degree that it allows its bearer to respond to the needs and feelings of others. Such knowledge is intuitive and holistic, and it is directly and preconsciously related to motivation and response. To analyse its content is to destroy it because this would remove it from that responsive comportment that is an essential part of it. The enemy of such feminine knowledge is masculine intellectualisation.

Liz and Gerry insisted that the dialogue had successfully uncovered knowledge of this form and was therefore as good as complete, while I felt that the important issues and the potentially transformative experience of understanding had not yet been broached. It seemed as if this disagreement was a particular instance of a larger debate arising from feminist critiques of western epistemology.

FEMINIST CRITIQUES OF WESTERN EPISTEMOLOGY

I decided to press Liz on the issue. What precisely was wrong with rational analysis and objective understanding? In reply, she suggested that the use of such rational and objective methods is precisely what is wrong with the way hospitals and other clinics are run. Patients are given numbers. They are objectified and reduced to their symptoms. Nursing work is rostered and timetabled in such a way as to jeopardise the opportunity for developing rapport with patients. Hospital administrations work to targets set by economic considerations and are driven by efficiency and cost-cutting. Nursing faculties in universities (Liz was a senior member of one of these) are similarly driven by economic-rationalist imperatives, with rising staff–student ratios, and privatisation of their research functions.

Although this was a familiar litany of complaints and one with which I could sympathise with readily enough, I did find it difficult to accept that this was all a masculine plot using the very forms of western reasoning for its nefarious purposes. It seemed more plausible to me to refer to this set of problems as a case of bureaucratic rationality rather than masculine rationality. Perhaps a fuller theoretical perspective on and critique of such rationality could derive from a thinker such as Jürgen Habermas, who refers to 'technocratic rationality' and sees it as expressing a deep-seated interest in technological control, whether of nature or of society (Habermas 1968). However this may be, it is certainly not obvious that such a rationality is distinctly male. There are plenty of women in positions of power in our hospital systems, who are just as adept at exercising such a form of rationality as their male counterparts. In any case, it is one of the burdens of Habermas' arguments that such forms of technocratic rationality are not expressions of the Enlightenment ideal. It is his concept of an 'emancipatory reason' that fully expresses this ideal, but our metadialogue was not the place to go into an elaborate theoretical exposition of these matters.

Liz was not one to accept my arguments without dispute. She was quick to point out that my point about female bureaucrats lacked intellectual rigour in that it was anecdotal and missed the point about the feminist critiques of western epistemology on which she was depending. The key point in these critiques is that the ideal subject of knowledge according to the Enlightenment ideal is a disembodied, deracinated, ahistorical, non-gendered and disinterested pure intellect. The traditional western epistemological subject engages in pure thought and debate from a position of objectivity and impartiality. He (and it usually is a 'he') occupies a 'view from nowhere' and creates knowledge that purports to be valid for 'anyone anywhere'. Examples of this kind of epistemological stance include the 'impartial spectator', the disinterested aesthetic gaze, the 'moral point of view', and 'value-free' science.

The only possible alternative to such a stance, according to the Enlightenment viewpoint, is relativism, with its claim that knowledge is nothing more than the point of view of the individual or community that proposes it. In this way lie obscurantism, superstition and all the epistemological evils of postmodernism.

Feminism has been at the forefront of the attack on this concept of knowledge (Alcoff and Potter 1993). In place of the abstracted epistemological subject, feminists have insisted on the concreteness and situatedness of knowers. That one is a woman, or black, or poor, or disabled, makes an important difference not only to what one knows but also to how one knows. That one is in relation with another, or belongs to an ethnic group, structures one's identity and, along with that, one's knowledge. To reject this as relativism is to beg the question whether such perspectival knowledge is valid. Every experience is fundamentally social, even the experience of experimental scientists in a laboratory. How much more so is the situational knowledge of nurses as they enter into relationships with patients and fellow workers? The argument is that, in rejecting the concrete situation of knowers, the Enlightenment ideal leaves us a form of knowledge that is systemically blind to what is most important to us as human beings.

There are those who would respond to this critique by saying that it proposes only a broadening of the bases of knowledge. They would say that it is valid to include intuition, situated insight, relational empathy and emancipatory interest in the sources of knowledge, but knowledge claims must still be evaluated and justified by using rigorous, objective, analytical, and rational means before they can be accepted as warranted. The feminist reply to this has been that, insofar as knowledge has practical importance in its application, knowledge claims should not be resolved just in the abstract. They should be evaluated not only as to their correspondence to facts but also as to their potential to enhance life and emancipate human beings from social and sexist oppression.

Once again it would take us too far afield to

adjudicate every aspect of this debate. The metadialogue had clearly become so theoretical and removed from the topic of the dialogue that nothing less than an academic study group could resolve the issues. One of the reasons that the Socratic dialogue method eschews theoretical discussions is that disagreements at this level become very readily intractable. When participants speak from their own experience and reality they have more chance of coming to agreement than if they speak from abstract positions that are based on ideologies or purely intellectual commitments. The quest for consensus requires participants to express themselves in terms that bear some authentic relation to their real experience and that allow others to enter sympathetically into that experience. What was happening here was that a philosophical debate had developed between Liz and myself while most of the others in the group were not participating.

Unfortunately, however, it became impossible to return to the main theme of the dialogue because time had run out. Even though Socratic dialogues take considerable time (often they are run over several days) the time allotted to this one had now ended and, perhaps to the relief of some, it had to end without a very satisfactory resolution.

A FINAL REFLECTION

Where does the Socratic dialogue method sit in the debate about knowledge that was raised in the metadialogue? The accusation was that it was on the side of masculinist, abstract, technocratic reason by virtue of its analytical and rational methods. I would want to defend it against this charge by making several brief points. First, it avoids the baneful effects of abstraction and objectivity because it stays close to real-life examples and authentic experience. Although it begins with a general question and its final phase (which was not reached on this occasion) opens up that question to its most general answers, it does so when group members have learned what it is most important to learn from the specific example that they have

discussed. Most of the time of the dialogue is spent exploring in meticulous detail the particularities of a specific incident. In this way, the Socratic and Enlightenment ideal of transformative understanding is realised by way of a discussion that has explored concrete and situated examples for most of the dialogue.

Secondly, the discussion takes place in a group that interacts very closely. There is no instance here of the abstracted and disembodied epistemological subject. Each participant in the dialogue is a real flesh and blood person with hopes, aspirations, disappointments and social relationships. It is from their own experience that they draw their examples and it is from their own experience (rather than theories and books) that they are asked to draw their contributions to the dialogue. In this they meet the feminist demand for a situated epistemological subject.

Thirdly, the dialogue is an activity of the group. It is not the activity of an isolated individual thinker. The insights that are won in the dialogue are won through discourse. Discourse is essentially a relation between the participants in the group. One gains understanding in a Socratic dialogue that one could not readily gain by oneself. One discovers new points of view and insights from the perspectives that others have. The relationships that one forms with others in the group (whether one agrees with them or not) contribute to the insights that one gains for oneself. The consensus towards which one is working requires that one listens and seeks to understand points of view with which one initially disagrees. It requires that one explain one's own point of view fully. This is not just cold and abstract analysis. It is an effort of communication. It is the other who is present with one in that room whom one is trying to convince and to whom one is trying to explain one's own perspective. This constitutes precisely the kind of interpersonal rapport that feminists have urged as the proper basis for valid knowledge. It is as important in dialogue to listen as it is to speak; one must remain open to the other. Assertions are offered as proposals open to revision rather than as claims to be defended. To explain oneself to another is not an act of domination. To convince another is not a conquest; it is a gift.

In summary, even though the Socratic dialogue method was developed historically in the light of the Enlightenment ideals of knowledge, it also instantiates the feminine and postmodern ways of knowing that stress the situatedness, holism and rapport of genuine insight. As a method of gaining knowledge it is fundamentally ethical.

REFERENCES

Alcoff L, Potter E (eds) 1993 Feminist epistemologies. Routledge, London

Carper B A 1978 Fundamental patterns of knowing in nursing. Advances in Nursing Science 1 (1): 13–24

Habermas J 1968 Erkenntnis und Interesse (Knowledge and Human Interests) (Shapiro J J trans 1987) Polity, Cambridge

van Hooft S 1999 Socratic dialogue as collegial reasoning. Practical Philosophy: Journal of the British Society of Consultant Philosophers 2 (2): 22–32

13

Creative approaches to ethics: poetry, prose and dialogue

Ann M. Begley

Some aspects of ethics will always be theoretical and analytical in content. However, Ann Begley makes a very strong point in this chapter that the immediate, raw, painful and contradictory aspects of lived experiences can never be based on theory, but can only be worked through at the moment. In order for health professionals to learn how to be with people in the situations when it hurts, literature, poetry, letters and accounts of dialogue come much nearer the reality. Ann gives examples of how such writing can be used in learning and teaching. These gems of literary art allow readers and students of every age to get right into a story. Beautifully crafted poetry or simple prose can give us insights that otherwise may never be possible. All we need to do is to listen and understand what is offered, but that in itself is an ethical act.

NURSING ETHICS: FROM OBEDIENCE TO COLLABORATION, FROM ETIQUETTE TO ETHICS

In 1962, Hilary Way suggested that: 'Matters of moral value fade imperceptibly into matters of etiquette…' (p. 14). The development of ethics as a subject in nursing has made considerable progress in the years since this book was written, particularly since the early 1990s. Extracts from books used in the not too distant past illustrate well how the role of the nurse has changed in relation to moral decision making. The professional nurse has, however, emerged as an autonomous moral agent who engages with other health care professionals and clients; collaboration and advocacy have replaced deference and blind obedience.

This is what was said then: 'Ward routine has a certain pattern to encourage respect for the doctor … he is never contradicted and, by various means, he is shown to be a person of pre-eminent skill and wisdom' (Way 1962, p. 22); and, if the doctor should make a mistake, 'in most cases we should obey the order and keep our eyes open for the consequences' (Way 1962, p. 22).

Today's nurses can scarcely believe that this perception of the nurse's role existed, but it is only in 1989 that this particular book on ethics for nurses was consigned to the archives (in one library at least!).

Another author illustrated how nurses were more concerned with etiquette than ethics:

The nurse must be prepared, however, to face the small-minded physicians when necessary. If she feels that a serious error has been made, her duty to her patient requires that she run the risk of an explosion from the doctor when she communicates with him. This danger can be reduced somewhat, even with the most irascible of physicians, if a tactful and respectful approach is made. Well chosen words, which subtly salve the ego of those who yearn for deference, may spell out the difference between good and bad feelings between physician and nurse (Denesford and Everett 1946, p. 161).

This was written at a time when nurses were expected to pledge to 'honour and obey the physician' (Garesche 1944, p. 300). This deference to the physician came before all other considerations, such as the physical welfare and moral input of the client.

Today this attitude is simply not acceptable; nurses are expected to question and collaborate rather than obey instructions. They are also expected to take on the role of advocacy. There is a definite shift in the perception of the nurse's role in moral decision making. Nurses who will practise far into this century will not be introduced to ethics from the perspective illustrated above. Students beginning their first semester now may still be practising in 2040. What new moral problems will they be faced with by that stage? Some recent developments, particularly in relation to reproductive technology, might have seemed like science fiction some years ago, but today's practitioner will be faced with dilemmas relating to such issues as human cloning. On the other hand, some moral problems, such as abortion and euthanasia, have been debated since the time of Hippocrates and even before then, yet these still present us with moral quandaries.

It is essential that nurses are able to explore these issues critically, that assertiveness, which was so lacking in the past, is fostered, and that the role of advocacy is approached with confidence, compassion and insight into the needs of clients.

As an academic subject, ethics has flourished in recent years, particularly in the education of health care professionals. In health care ethics the appropriateness of the principle-based approach (Beauchamp and Childress 1989) and traditional moral theory (consequentialism and deontology) have been questioned. Some have proposed a shift in focus, suggesting that, for example, an ethic of care or virtue theory are more appropriate approaches to health care ethics. Traditional moral theory was challenged in 1958 by Elizabeth Anscombe and subsequently by Alastair MacIntyre (1985). These and others now pose a serious threat in their attempt to oust traditional theories that are based on concepts such as duty, obligation and principles; those who use these approaches to ethics (which still form the diet of most ethics programmes in nursing) are being challenged by these 'newer', less objective ideas.

The chapters in this book reflect the widening array of approaches to ethics with which today's practitioners are presented. Debates relating to theoretical approaches will continue, but we need to remember when preparing students for practice, and when facilitating ongoing educational support for practitioners, that they are not philosophy students; we are concerned with applied ethics, not meta-ethics. For this reason and, in addition to introducing nurses to normative (or substantive ethics), a practical approach, in which the issues are considered from the client's perspective, is needed. At the same time, heightening nurses' sensitivity to clients' needs is essential. How can we achieve this?

A PRACTICAL APPROACH: LITERATURE, DIALOGUE AND ETHICS

We need to nurture insight (the power of seeing into and understanding things: imaginative penetration) into the lives of others; this is essential for a sensitive approach to moral problems in real life. If we want practitioners to achieve this when they are involved in moral problems, we must ensure that they are given an opportunity to apply theory to the world of experience. All practitioners do not have an identical range of past experience. Some will have experienced bereavement, some will even have had an opportunity to care for a dying relative or friend, while others will not. We cannot, however, arrange for students to have experience of, for example, death and miscarriage. We can tell them about the emotions people feel, and we can discuss research findings, but we cannot arrange for them to feel these emotions themselves. They may feel unable really to empathise with someone owing to their own lack of experience and insight. A more imaginative approach for practitioners and clinical mentors, however, could facilitate the development of the insight necessary to understand patients' experiences and problems in a real way. This opportunity to experience is essential for the development of an understanding of the individual whose life is affected by our moral judgement, that is, for moral sensitivity. The problem that arises from an inability to offer real life experience may be resolved to some extent by the use of literature and vicarious experience (Begley 1996).

LITERATURE AND ETHICS

Today, many people (Begley 1995, 1996, Downie and Calman 1987) suggest that literature can help to cultivate the different and deeper type of understanding that nurses need. Robin Downie and Kenneth Calman (1987, p. 36–37) refer to this as 'vertical understanding'. Understanding in this sense is gained through looking at the 'named individual now standing in front of us' and acquiring insight into the 'individual personal history'. This is different from scientific or horizontal understanding, which is more concerned with general principles and the typical patient rather than the unique individual. Downie and Calman use the German word verstehen to describe understanding 'of the kind we aim at when we try to put ourselves on the inside of the actions of others and capture their meaning for them'. Literature helps us to explore these unique situations, to 'capture the meaning' that the experience has for the other person, and to empathise. Literature can, through a process of 'sensitising sympathy', lead us to real emotional awareness and ultimately to compassion, the term that Downie and Calman use to express 'imaginative and sensitised sympathy.'

Wisdom from the Greeks

Since before the time of Plato and Aristotle, the value of literature has been a source of discussion and argument (Begley 1996). According to Plato (427–347 BC), the arts, particularly poetry, were an imitation of reality or *mimesis*: a copying of real life by means of literature and the visual arts. Plato considered poetry to be valuable as a means of evoking 'pity and fear' (Dorsch 1988, p. 14). The effect of poetry on people, and its capacity to bring about an emotional response, was also recognised by Aristotle (384–322 BC), who commented that 'these poets may succeed wonderfully in getting the effect they want, that is, one which is tragic and appeals to our humanity'(Dorsch 1988, p. 14).

Plato used the Dialogues to elucidate many questions of a moral nature and these writings illustrate well how dialogue can be used to convey reality and insight. In the Dialogues, he uses an aporetic approach, which does not necessarily commit either Socrates or himself to any of the views expressed (Irwin 1976, p. 6). The modern reader of the Platonic Dialogues will not find conclusive answers to the themes emerging from the discussions of the interlocutors. MacIntyre (1985) suggests that Socrates was not really attempting to secure a conclusion; he was, rather, trying to achieve a change in the hearers. This is an interesting point and it is of immense interest today. The modern writer of dialogue may well employ this method to challenge beliefs; it is useful when the intention is to present conflicting views in a convincing way. Like Plato, the writer of a dialogue can raise issues and proffer resolutions to problems by the use of characters, without having to support one view over the other. It is an excellent method for exploring dilemmas, both for individual readers and for group activity and discussion.

Creative literature, vicarious experience and moral judgement

Is experience, vicarious or otherwise, important in moral decision making? According to Aristotle, wisdom is excellence in theoretical matters, and excellence in practical matters is called practical wisdom (phronesis) (see Ch. 2). Practical wisdom entails the ability to plan one's life well; we need deliberation and to be in control (Urmson 1998). The scope of practical wisdom is limited to excellence in deliberation and we need experience for understanding and being able to interpret situations; therefore, maturity is required. For theoretical excellence, on the other hand, we do not need this experience. For example, a nurse who has recently passed examinations and registered for the first time as a qualified professional will be competent in certain elements of nursing care. The more experienced nurse, having both theoretical excellence and years of appropriate practice, would have more insight and therefore an ability to anticipate complications. We also need 'cleverness' for practical wisdom and this enables us to execute our plans.

The 'new' nurse with an excellent memory may not be 'clever' in this other sense. Having passed examinations does not guarantee that he or she has the ability to use theoretical knowledge to make sound judgements, to act appropriately, or, in other words, to be a 'good nurse'. Practical wisdom enables us to know the means to the end and also to know which ends are worthy. We cannot have excellence of character (moral virtue) without practical wisdom or practical wisdom without excellence of character.

In Aristotle's approach, ethics is portrayed as knowledge of particulars, not knowledge of universals. 'Good' is ambiguous and we cannot claim that it is a universal. In particular circumstances there is no general rule by which we can decide on the right course of action. This is one reason why so many people are beginning to question traditional moral theory and a principle-based approach to ethics. There are complexities in real life and there could be no simple rule to deal with all events. There are important general principles, but, according to Aristotle and those who advocate a virtue theoretical approach to health care ethics, we cannot use these to determine the 'mean' on particular occasions.

'Now questions of conduct and expedience have as little fixety about them as questions of what is healthful; and if this is true of the general rule, it is still more true that its application to particular problems admits of no precision' (Aristotle NE 1103b26–30, 1970 rev trans p. 93).

If we accept Aristotle's position then it is clear that the more experience the nurse has, the more insight will be gained not only into clients' perspectives and clinical practice, but also into how to act appropriately. Anne Scott (1995) highlights how Aristotle's emphasis on practice will 'strike a chord' with practitioners and students, but, as already noted, it is not always possible to gain certain experiences through practice; we must sometimes rely on vicarious experience to fill the gap.

Vicarious experience is not experienced personally but imagined through reading about or observing the experience of others. Although the situations to which we respond are imaginary, the felt emotions are real. Today's modern fiction can have an equally potent effect on the emotions. A book, poem or dialogue can move an individual to laugh or cry in response to the fiction. Literature has the power to bring about strong emotional responses in an unreal situation. The reader becomes involved in the experience, rather than simply remaining in the audience (Begley 1995, 1996). Nurses need this level of insight. They need to get right into the story if they are to approach people with compassion and moral sensitivity.

In addition to dialogue there is a vast range of literature, such as novels, poetry and letters, which can be used to help nurses to develop insight into real-life tragedy and human suffering. It is difficult to think of situations that have not been written about. Practitioners could be encouraged to make their own contribution to a clinically-based, or ward-based, collection of material and an ethics interest group could come together to discuss problems encountered and to exchange useful material. Nurses could be encouraged to be creative, to write of their encounters and to give an account of their discussions with patients or debates with other staff. Everyday conversations are charged with issues for discussion; we only have to listen!

LITERATURE, ETHICS AND INSIGHT: SELECTED EXAMPLES

A novel: death and dying

A novella such as Tolstoy's *Death of Ivan Ilych* (1886) helps us really to move into the experiences of a dying person. Isolation, fear, frustration and anger overcame the dying man and Tolstoy clearly describes how he felt when faced with his own immortality: 'Anger choked him and he was agonizingly, unbearably, miserable' (p. 258).

Tolstoy highlights how nurses and other health care professionals may be so caught up in technology and pharmacology that the value of simple, comforting remedies, which the patient finds helpful, are underestimated and often ignored. Ivan Ilych found that his medication was of little use but that his pain was relieved by having his legs raised for long periods. A peasant boy who cared for him often sat all night supporting his master's legs on his shoulders, while the doctor sneered at this approach. The despair and loneliness felt by Ivan Illych is obvious in the following words: 'He wept on account of his helplessness, his terrible loneliness, the cruelty of God, the absence of God' (p. 271).

This 50-page novella can help us to gain insight into the often tragic results of a lack of communication, and the fear and isolation that can arise out of this. Ivan Ilych lost the fear of death in his last few hours, but the reader is left with the feeling that, even though 'in the place of death there was light' (p. 279), this person still died feeling abandoned and left to face the challenge of dying alone. He died still feeling that he was a nuisance to his family, and detached from those around him: '"It is finished!" said someone near to him. He heard these words and repeated them in his soul. "Death is finished", he said to himself. "It is no more!"' (p. 279).

The death, or rather the dying process, of Ivan Ilych caused destruction within the family. This can happen in real life and this novel can help us to see into this type of situation. It can also provide an introduction to the discussion of the wider professional and moral issues arising in the care of terminally ill people, such as truth telling. There is, for example, a lack of frank discussion of Ivan's illness and prognosis. Doctors are arrogant, there is a veil of secrecy and no consideration of client autonomy.

A poem – miscarriage and stillbirth

Seamus Heaney (1969) wrote of miscarriage with moving sensitivity. In *Elegy for a Still Born Child* the poet describes the intense sense of loss felt by the woman (who has had a spontaneous abortion) and her husband.

The woman, having become accustomed to the movement, the presence within her, is now unlearning the familiar movements of the fetus and, in her grief, she becomes 'heavy' with a feeling of 'lightness'. The poem expresses the excitement and then the disappointment of her husband. He had watched the growth and anticipated eagerly the birth of his first child.

The sadness, the pain, and the feeling of irreplaceable loss and confusion are expressed in the following lines:

A wreath of small clothes, a memorial pram,
and parents reaching for a phantom limb (p. 32).

Through such imagery, nurses and midwives could be drawn into the experiences of people in these circumstances. It is often implied that a stillborn child is replaceable; it is simply a matter of having another child. The poem helps us to appreciate, however, that this child was unique and the loss was similar to the loss of a limb; the phantom limb will continue to cause pain and will not be easily forgotten.

Literature, therefore, can provide a window through which we can see into the experiences of others. An introduction to literature such as this can enhance nurses' ability to perceive the needs of these people in real life and, ultimately, to promote empathy and a more sensitive approach to moral decision making and care in general.

Experiences of death and dying, miscarriage and birth have always been part of our human experience and are sometimes referred to as 'old moral problems', as opposed to 'new moral problems', such as those arising from recent advances in reproductive technology. Human reproduction is fraught with moral problems, and the midwives and nurses of today face the challenge of dilemmas generated by technological advances. Examples of these are fetal egg donation, cadaver egg donation, preimplantation diagnosis, and posthumous parenting (Harris and Holm 1998). The following examples, a letter and a dialogue, highlight the problems that some nurses and midwives may have to face in the future. Unlike the previous examples of Tolstoy and Heaney, these extracts are from works that have been written with the express purpose of raising philosophical and ethical questions through a literary medium.

A LETTER: FROM A POSTMENOPAUSAL MOTHER TO HER TEENAGE DAUGHTER

Inez de Beaufort (1998) gives us some insight into the problems faced by a couple whose child was conceived using this new technology. She does this by means of a letter written by a 'postmenopausal' mother to her daughter. The method used is powerful; the reader almost feels embarrassed and there is a sense of discomfort, as if we are prying into someone's private life and correspondence. The letter expresses the hurt of the birth mother and father, and the shame of their daughter. Issues such as the problem of identifying the genetic mother are raised. The birth mother speaks directly to her daughter and we, the readers, are left wondering how her daughter will react; we are perhaps even hoping that she will be sensitive to her mother's distress and the obvious pain and love.

For your eighteenth birthday, this milestone of adulthood, I'm writing you this letter. A plea for the accused? An explanation for more understanding, if need be posthumously? A justification? A testament for later, for when you are in a more reflective mood?…I've never known what to do with your shame… There is a lot you can reproach me with, but not that I've acted on impulse. Parents who are trying to have children for thirty years don't do that out of frivolity; they have thought too much about it rather than too little…Young as I was then – sorry for the cynicism, I still thought that I could influence the prejudices. But we were execrated by our wholesome fellow men. We gave interviews, appeared in numerous talk shows on television. The modern but scarcely more humane alternative to the freak show. From the fattest lady of the country to one of the oldest mothers of the country. Let's gaze and judge (p. 238–247).

When some new moral problem arises it generally causes a sensation. The front pages of the newspapers report the latest development and quite often the women who are the subject of these reports are vilified, or at least portrayed as superficial and selfish. The issues raised are then discussed by students studying ethics, by practitioners, in academic circles and literature. People and situations become abstract and the people concerned have no real opportunity to give their side of the story. How could an introduction to the real person affect our perceptions of the woman and her family? de Beaufort's letter raises the moral problems discussed in academic articles, newspapers and textbooks, but these take on a different light when presented to the reader as a first-person account of the experience of the family involved. It also raises the issue of prejudice. Nurses have their own prejudices, and, even though they are professionally obliged to refrain from acting on these or showing them (and most are able to do so), they can still stifle empathy and influence moral judgement.

DIALOGUE AND ETHICS

Another of the many complex moral issues arising from reproductive technology and one with which midwives and nurses are faced more frequently, is that of multifetal pregnancy reduction. The issues are here discussed from three perspectives, the pregnant woman and her partner (clients), and a midwife. The medium used to highlight the problems faced by these characters is a dialogue. This is done in an attempt to introduce a degree of reality and foster insight into the feelings of the clients. It is presented as an example of how this approach can bring ethics to life for the practitioner (Begley 2000). In the Platonic dialogues, Socrates engaged in discussion with many different characters and these characters were used to represent different 'sides' of the argument. As mentioned above, this approach is a useful way of presenting a variety of views without committing oneself to any of them. It is certainly very useful for a teacher who wishes to explore complex issues and facilitate discussion in health care.

The following dialogue is taken from *Nursing Ethics* 2000 7(2) and is reproduced by kind permission of the publisher, Arnold, London (Begley 2000, p. 102–109).

Clare and John have been trying to start a family for 10 years. Clare has had fertility treatment and she now has a positive pregnancy test. They are very excited and are anxiously awaiting an ultrasound scan.

Clare: It's hard to believe, isn't it – a human being, a tiny person – a boy or a girl? For some strange reason, call it intuition, I feel strongly that this is a boy…

John: Maybe two if we're lucky – a boy and a girl! It won't be long before they can tell us what the sex is; maybe even in a few more weeks.

Clare: I don't really want to be told, do you?

John: It might be better to wait and to have something to look forward to, but I don't know if I'll be able to resist the temptation of asking! A son or daughter – you're right, it is hard to believe. I used to think that people were a bit daft going all emotional about pregnancy before there was even a bump, but I understand now.

Clare: Yes, and I'm surprised at how responsible and protective I feel. Everything I do, everything I eat and drink, is weighed up and considered in relation to the effect on this baby. It's a strange feeling – like your body and lifestyle has been hijacked; but it is not an unpleasant feeling.

John: How are we going to wait another seven or eight months?

Clare: It'll go by quickly enough – we've got a lot of preparation – nursery, equipment, clothes…

John: Hold on there! We've a few months to go before we start all that, but I suppose I'm really looking forward to it; after all, we've waited for a long time for this moment – we'll enjoy every minute of it.

Clare: I suppose we shouldn't get carried away with plans and be so wrapped up in excitement that we aren't prepared for the possibility of there being something wrong, or that something may happen…

John: Something like what? What could happen?

Clare: All right! Don't panic! I'm just afraid to feel too happy and secure because I am afraid of being disappointed.

John: We'll take one step at a time. We've got the scan in the morning. Have you ever seen the pictures from a scan? They're fantastic! Jim brought his baby's scan into work to let us see. I have to admit that I thought him a bit 'soft' at the time, but I feel different now. Did you know that we can have a video made of the scan, and that you can see the baby move, even

sometimes sucking its thumb and… what's so funny?

Clare: And you thought that Jim had gone soft? Listen to yourself!

John: I wonder if it can hear us talking. Will it know our voices when it is born?

Clare: I think that eight weeks is a bit soon for that, but maybe he can. Anyway, I'm exhausted – save your enthusiasm for tomorrow!

The next day: after the scan

Sandra is an experienced midwife but this is her first encounter with people facing this type of dilemma.

Midwife: Are you sure that there is nothing I can get you? What about your husband – should I go and look for him?

Clare: No, thanks, he'll be back when he calms down.

Midwife: I'm sorry – I'm just concerned about him. I'll wait with you. I don't know what to say except that you can talk to me now if you want to, but you can come back at any time if you prefer.

Clare: I'm sorry for snapping. I just can't take it in. Yesterday we were so happy, and today the whole thing has just exploded in our faces. Three or four babies would have been a shock, but we would have welcomed them… it's as if we've got everything and nothing at the same time. It's like winning the lottery and losing the ticket. I've got seven babies and at the same time I have none. What happens now? What can we do?

Midwife: The obstetrician will come and discuss the options with you when John returns, unless you would prefer to see him alone.

Clare: No! We need to talk about this together. I don't know where he has gone – he didn't say a word.

One hour later John returns and the obstetrician explains that the likelihood of Clare carrying seven fetuses to term is extremely slim. The option most likely to ensure a live birth is reduction of the multifetal pregnancy, although this procedure does carry risks. Clare is advised that she should consider reducing the pregnancy to two or three fetuses. The procedure is explained to the couple and they discuss their position when the obstetrician leaves. Clare asks the midwife to stay with them in case they need further clarification and because she senses that she is 'tuned in' to their predicament.

At home

John: We were so happy last night. We actually joked about the possibility of having twins. I had a feeling that it was too good to last.

Clare: What are we going to do?

John: I don't know. One minute I agree with the doctor, the next minute I'm thinking how can we deliberately choose two or three out of the seven and kill the others?

Clare: That's the problem. I don't think that we can choose. Yesterday when I thought that I only had one baby I felt so close to it. I even thought of it as a boy. Now I know that I've got seven, I don't think that I can suddenly start thinking of them as disposable 'things'.

John: But they're not babies yet – they're just bundles of cells and…

Clare: Yesterday you were so excited that you wanted to take a video. You wondered if it could hear our voices and you talked about your son or daughter as a little person! Now that there is a problem they're just bundles of cells. They have as much right to live as you or I…

John: Don't be angry with me. I'm trying to make it easier for us. If we think of the seven as human beings….

Clare: Of course they're human beings. They're our babies…

John: But they haven't got personalities. They're not people, or persons in their own right yet…

Clare: They will be if we give them a chance…

John: But that's the point! They won't; none of them will have the chance if we try to keep them all! We have to sacrifice some so that others will survive! …

Clare: I'm sorry, I can't accept that. We can't kill four for the sake of three. As far as I'm concerned it's either all or nothing. I don't think that we could live with the guilt of having deliberately killed four or five of our babies.

John: But if they all die then will we not feel guilty about the ones who could have been saved? Is it not worse to let seven babies die than to kill four and save three?

Clare: But that's out of our hands. If it happens, then that is letting nature take its course. We can't be responsible for that.

John: Would we not be responsible for *not preventing* it?

Clare: I don't know if I could be happy if I did this. I don't think that I could ever justify deliberately killing some to ensure that others survive… The end doesn't justify the means. They're all innocent. Anyway, there's no guarantee that having done this the others will survive.

John: Yes, but they are more likely to. And what about your own health? We have to think about the risk of trying to carry all the babies. We aren't taking lives without a good reason. Our intention is to save life. Surely that justifies termination? …

Clare: It's too soon to make a decision. We need time to think, but I'm fairly certain that I'll take the risk and try to keep all of them.

John: Yes, but we'll probably lose them all.

Clare: But the point I'm making is that it is possible that they will survive – maybe all of them. If we lose some at birth, then at least we know that we've given them the best chance available. If we kill some now, we will never get over the guilt; at least I won't.

John: But hundreds of women have abortions every day. Are you saying that they're guilty of murdering babies?

Clare: Don't put words into my mouth. Of course I'm not saying that. The point is that we want this pregnancy. We planned it and now we've got to select some for life and some for death. Women have abortions for all sorts of reasons. It's the only option for many. I don't believe that this is the only option for us. Other women have different values and we can't judge them, but I could never consider abortion under any circumstances.

John: Not even if there was a serious deformity in a baby, or if there was a major risk to your own life? So far, all of these babies seem fine but what if another scan shows that three of them have deformities? Would you not consider it then? What if there is a major risk to your own life? I'm not happy about taking the risk. I still think that we should listen to the experts.

Clare: What experts? Doctors are no more experts in this than we are! As far as I'm concerned, we have a fifty-fifty chance of success. Doctors and midwives are experts, but they're not moral experts. They're no more able to decide what we should do than we are. They can advise us on the risks, but they can't decide for us.

John: I don't think that abortion is right in most circumstances, but there are certain situations when it seems to be the only option.

Clare: You're contradicting yourself. You either agree that abortion is wrong or you agree that it's right. You can't justify it by saying that you're doing it to save lives; you can't justify a morally unacceptable act by pointing to good consequences…

John: You seem to have made up your mind. Have I got no say in this? What if I lose you and all of these babies? What if this pregnancy causes damage and you are unable to have more children?

Clare: We can go on saying 'what if?' for ever and it won't make any difference because I can't make a decision to *do* anything. We'll just have to wait and see what happens. We don't have to do anything for another three or four weeks; we've time to think. I don't think that I'll change my mind but the midwife said that we could ring at any time, or call in.

The midwife's thoughts

Sandra is more acutely aware than ever before that a real dilemma is unfolding. She has always felt pretty safe in her own moral beliefs, but for the first time she is really involved and feels that her moral convictions are being shaken. As Clare and John discuss the problem in their own words, Sandra recalls discussion of these issues in ethics classes. She thought that she could apply theory easily to practice but finds this more difficult in the real situation. Somehow or other, an appeal to objective principles and theory does not offer the insight needed in a situation like this. The dialogue raises the following issues. (Although the discussion focuses on the moral status of the fetus, nurses face similar problems when caring for people with, for example, persistent vegetative state.)

Personhood

Many people use the words 'person' and 'human being' interchangeably, considering them to be one and the same thing. In health care ethics this issue arises often in relation to ethics at the beginning of life (midwifery) and to ethics at the end of life (nursing). Being biologically human is considered to be the only criterion necessary for being a person. Others, however, believe that there is a significant difference between the concepts 'human being' and 'person'. Human being is a biological concept, while person is more concerned with values. This is very much reflected in Heaney's poem, where values were more to the fore than biological considerations.

In the dialogue there appears to be a degree of ambivalence and certainly a clash of values in relation to the moral status of the fetus. Clare has no doubts that the fetuses are persons; John used the term loosely when things were going well, but reverted to the biological concept of the fetus when a problem arose.

Argument from potential

Clare appeals to the argument from potential and claims that we should respect a fetus because of the person it will become. Although a fetus is a *potential* person, it is not an *actual* person (Harris 1983).

Principle of utility

John is employing the principle of utility. He is carrying out a utilitarian calculation: there will be four dead fetuses, but the termination opens up the possibility of a much longed for 'ready-made family'. John believes (or at least tries to convince himself) that it is acceptable to terminate four embryos in favour of three. The alternative is the possibility that all fetuses will abort spontaneously and this, according to John, is an outcome that should be avoided if possible.

Absolute principles

Clare believes in the absolute prohibition on killing the innocent and the Kantian maxim that one should not use others as a means to an end. Killing four to save three would be using them as a means to an end. Clare's moral appraisal of termination, unlike John's, does not involve any consideration of the consequences. She does not believe that 'the end justifies the means'.

Letting die and killing

Clare believes that 'letting nature take its course' and doing nothing is more morally acceptable than taking positive action that leads to death. John is clear that he considers it to be morally justifiable to sacrifice four for the greater good because three have more chance of survival than all seven. Clare thinks differently; she is more optimistic and, while there is a strong possibility that she will lose all of the babies, this is by no means certain.

The midwife

Sandra has not felt prepared by her ethics education for the feeling of powerlessness felt by those on the horns of a true dilemma. Listening to the discussion of the parents in this case has shaken her confidence in her previous convictions. She has always shared Clare's strong absolutist approach to issues such as abortion and multifetal pregnancy reduction. She considers the deliberate ending of life to be absolutely morally wrong. Sandra considered the fetus to be more than a biological entity. According to her views, the fetus is a person; it therefore has rights and, in circumstances such as refused caesarean section, Sandra would claim that the fetus should be protected from harm or death even if this means overriding maternal autonomy. She considers it to be a question of a balance between the principles of beneficence (to do good) and non-maleficence (to do no harm). She, like Clare, is guided by the absolute prohibition on deliberately killing innocent persons. Sandra now feels differently about multifetal embryo reduction. This is because there is not only the issue of the rights of *one* fetus competing with maternal rights, but in this case one must consider the rights of *some* fetuses competing with the rights of other fetuses. This is a problem for her. Not having the pregnancy reduced could leave seven dead, while having the pregnancy reduced would definitely kill four but leave a better opportunity for three to live. In other words, doing nothing (omission) can result in a seemingly worse outcome than acting. More importantly, Sandra's moral stance has been shaken by being right in there with the parents. She is finding it impossible to take an objective position. The utilitarian calculus and the Kantian notion of obligation and duty somehow or other seem to be wanting. Experience has altered her perception of the situation and made her more sensitive to the context and values.

As with any moral dilemma, there is no straightforward answer. No option emerges clearly as the most morally acceptable. The couple represented in the dialogue share one overwhelming desire: to have a healthy child or children. Whatever their decision, they will not both be happy. Midwives and nurses have a crucial role to play in this sort of scenario. It is often difficult for people to reconcile their own moral positions with the responsibility of supporting the client, whatever his or her choice or the outcome of that choice.

The nature of professional ethics has changed so much in the last two decades that nurses now find it difficult to believe that the books quoted earlier were ever taken seriously. Today's professionals need to be prepared to face problems that were the stuff of science fiction some years ago; for this they need experience, if not real, then imaginary. It is my belief that the approaches described above can best feed the imagination. Whether the problems faced are 'old' or 'new', nurses and midwives need to be aware of the need for experience, real or vicarious. Whatever the theoretical framework used to help to resolve moral problems, be it from within the perspective of traditional moral theory, virtue ethics or caring ethics, they will be better placed to make judgements if they have some insight into the real-life experiences of clients. A creative approach using literature and dialogue is one way in which this can be achieved.

REFERENCES

Anscombe G E M 1958 Modern moral philosophy. Philosophy 33 (124): 1–19

Aristotle. In: Thompson J A K (trans) rev 1970 The ethics of Aristotle; the Nicomachean ethics. Penguin, Harmondsworth, p. 93

Beauchamp T L, Childress J F 1989 Principles of biomedical ethics, 3rd edn. Oxford University Press, New York

Begley A M 1995 Literature, ethics and the communication of insight. Nursing Ethics 2 (4): 288–294

Begley A M 1996 Literature and poetry: pleasure and practice. International Journal of Nursing Practice 2 (4): 182–188

Begley A M 2000 Preparation for practice in the new millennium: a discussion of the moral implications of multifetal pregnancy reduction. Nursing Ethics 7 (2): 99–112

de Beaufort I 1998 Letter from a postmenopausal mother. In: Harris J, Holm S (eds) 1998 The future of human reproduction. Oxford University Press, New York, p. 238–247

Denesford K J, Everett M S 1946 Ethics for modern nurses. Saunders, Philadelphia, PA

Dorsch T 1988 Introduction to classical literary criticism: Aristotle, Horace, Longinus. Penguin, London

Downie R, Calman K C 1987 Healthy respect: ethics in health care. Faber and Faber, London, p. 36–38

Garesche E F 1944 Ethics and the art of conduct for nurses, 2nd edn. Saunders, Philadelphia, PA

Harris J 1983 In vitro fertilization; the ethical issues. Philosophical Quarterly 33 (132): 218–237

Harris J, Holm S (eds) 1998 The future of human reproduction. Oxford University Press, New York

Heaney S 1969 Elegy for a still born child. In: Door into the dark. Faber and Faber, London, p. 31–32

Irwin T 1976 Plato's moral theories. Oxford University Press, Oxford

MacIntyre A 1985 After virtue: a study in moral theory, 2nd edn. Duckworth, London, p. 121–164

Scott P A 1995 Aristotle, nursing and health care ethics. Nursing Ethics 2 (4): 279–285

Tolstoy L 1886 The death of Ivan Ilych. (Maude L, Maude A trans 1906) In: The raid and other stories. Oxford University Press, Oxford 1986 World Classic Edition, p. 228–278

Urmson J O 1998 Aristotle's ethics. Blackwell, Oxford

Way H 1962 Ethics for nurses. Macmillan, London

Further reading

Aristotle. In: Thompson J A K trans rev 1976. The ethics of Aristotle; the Nicomachean ethics. Penguin, Harmondsworth

Plato. In: Hamilton H, Cairns H (eds) 1994. The collected dialogues of Plato. Princeton University Press, Princeton, NJ

Index